MW00825249

Guidebook to
Ace the Lifestyle Medicine Boards

Figures and Tables for Easy Study

Nupur Garg, M.D., DipABLM

Jessica Lee, M.D., DipABLM

Acknowledgements
For contributions to the content, we are grateful to Shirlee Kuhl, MD, FAAP, DipABLM and Keegan Ziemba, MD, MPH, DipABLM.
For his assistance with copyediting and formatting, we are grateful to Peter Heytler.
For support and encouragement throughout the process, we are grateful to Eben Olson and Richard Lee.

Inquiries
The authors intend to update this book for quality and completeness. If after completing the book, you would like to provide corrections, comments, or contributions, please email us at guideaceLMexam@gmail.com. Entries will be reviewed, and significant contribution will be compensated at the discretion of the authors. If your submission is used in future versions, you will receive a personal acknowledgement plus a $10 Amazon gift card. All contributions will become property of the authors and are subject to editing. Please include a reference if applicable.

Disclaimer
This book reflects our knowledge as it pertains to passing the ABLM exam. This book is not meant to be used in any other way. The authors have reviewed the information carefully and checked with sources to be reliable in their effort to provide accurate and up-to-date information. We do not guarantee that anything in this book is factual in perpetuity as new knowledge is constantly being created. There is also the possibility of human error that could have occurred at many stages during the compilation of this book. We advise each person to verify for themselves that the information in this book is accurate and complete before using the contents of this book in a clinical setting.

Publisher: JSN LLC
ISBN: 979-8-9863663-1-9
Copyright ©2024 JSN LLC
All rights reserved

TABLE OF CONTENTS

CHAPTER ONE
WELCOME

Congratulations on choosing this book as your guide to ACE the Lifestyle Medicine Exam! Every author and contributor to this book has taken and passed the American Board of Lifestyle Medicine (ABLM) Exam. We thoroughly enjoyed the material, but we preferred this format for digesting it (pun intended). We think you will too!

Historically, the ABLM/IBLM exam has a high pass rate. While that may be reassuring, if you are planning on practicing in Lifestyle Medicine or have any interest in integrating it into your practice, then learning the information thoroughly is a great reason to take the exam seriously. If, by the time you've reached the end of your studying journey, you felt that we left anything out, we would like to invite you to give us feedback. Please reach out at GuideAceLMexam@gmail.com.

Overview of Pathway to Become Diplomate ABLM/IBLM (ABLM Certification)
The requirements to become a certified diplomate of ABLM/IBLM vary based on your professional category, your residential location, and the pathway to certification that you have chosen. The following steps outline the most common pathway:

1. Register to become an American College of Lifestyle Medicine (ACLM) member (do this first to get discounts on the rest of the steps). Note: You do not have to be a member of ACLM to take the exam.
2. Register to take the ABLM exam.
3. Purchase and complete the Fundamentals of LM Board Review course from ACLM or Lifestyle Medicine Core Competencies. (You need to buy the version with CME unless you have another plan for fulfilling the CME requirements for becoming an ACLM/ICLM diplomate.)
4. Attend the ACLM conference or other approved conferences to get the in-person CME.
5. Complete the case report (see FAQs below).
6. Upload required documents and certificates on the ABLM website.
7. Take the exam.

Unless you have discounts for other sources of CME or do the residency/fellowship pathway for completing requirements to become a certified diplomate, these steps are currently the cheapest and most straightforward way to get certified. That said, the total costs will still be slightly more than $3,000.

Important Dates and Timeline
Registration for the exam closes end of September
The certification exam is typically held late November/early December
Exam results are posted end of December

Pre-requisites
1. 30 online CME (from ablm.org/eligibility-prerequisites)
     - ACLM Foundations of Lifestyle Medicine Board Review Course
     - ACLM/ACPM Lifestyle Medicine Core Competencies (LMCC)
     - Doane University Lifestyle Medicine Professional Certificate Program
     - Weill Cornell Medicine – Qatar, Certificate in Lifestyle Medicine
     - Universidad Abierta Interamericana (Argentina) – Academic Diploma in Lifestyle Medicine (in Spanish)
     - Diplomado de Medicina del Estilo de Vida (Chile- en español) Universidad del Desarrollo- Sociedad Chilena de Medicina del estilo de Vida (SOCHIMEV)
     - LifestylePro Academy Életmódorvos szakmai továbbképzés (Lifestyle Medicine Physician continuing education)
     - LifestylePro Academy Életmódszakértő szakmai továbbképzés (Lifestyle Medicine Professional continuing education)

2. 20 in-person OR virtual CME
     - ACLM annual conference
     - International Plant Based Nutrition Healthcare Annual Conferences
     - Plant-based Prevention of Disease (P-POD) Annual Conferences
     - PCRM Annual International Conferences on Nutrition in Medicine
     - Annual AAFP Lifestyle Medicine course
     - Weill Cornell Medicine – Qatar, Certificate in Lifestyle Medicine
     - Harvard Annual LM conference: Tools for Promoting Healthy Change

3. Case report – FAQs:
     - *What are the specifications of the case report?*
There is a pdf of the outline here: https://ablm.org/wp-content/uploads/2023/01/MDDOCertificationCaseStudyTemplate-1.pdf

     - *Are there any other tools for guidance available?*
It helps to go through the Key Clinical Processes chapter and then the chapter on the pillar related to the intervention you prescribed.

     - *Can you use yourself?*
Yes, in fact we believe most case reports are about oneself.

     - *Are there any existing examples?*
We don't know of any examples publicly available.

     - *Has anyone's case report ever been rejected?*
Not that we know of.

     - *Is there a word limit?*
We suggest writing at least 200 words for the Reflections section, but we do not think you need much more.

- Any other advice?
We believe that this pre-requisite is more of a check mark than anything graded. Don't stress too much. If you follow the outline provided, you should be fine.

Understanding the Exam and this Guidebook
Exam Logistics:
- One block of exam questions
- 150 questions for physicians; 120 questions for practitioners
- 240 minutes
- Located at Prometric testing centers (the last two years had virtual options)
- Americans with Disability Act-approved accommodations are available (email ABLM directly)
- Nursing mothers' accommodations available (email ABLM directly)

Table 1-1. Exam Breakdown and Competencies

Topic	Percentage on Exam	Number of Questions (150)
Introduction to Lifestyle Medicine	4%	6
Fundamentals of Health Behavior Change	10%	15
Key Clinical Processes in Lifestyle Medicine	8%	12
The Role of Physician Health and Physician's Personal Health	4%	6
Nutrition Science, Assessment, and Prescription	26%	39
Physical Activity Science and Prescription	14%	21
Emotional and Mental Well-Being, Assessment, and Interventions	10%	15
Sleep Health Science and Interventions	8%	12
Managing Tobacco Cessation and Other Toxic Exposure	8%	12
The Role of Connectedness and Positive Psychology	8%	12

(Source: ABLM website)

The topics above are broken down further into core competencies (see fusionwebservice.com/ablm/lifestyle-medicine-core-competencies/). Each test question falls under one or more of these core competencies. We have primarily relied upon Tables and Figures, but you will see other kinds of formats as well, like a breakdown on how to handle certain exam questions. In addition, the Key Studies have changed over the years; be sure to obtain the most recent list.

Sources Used Throughout this Book

Agency for Healthcare Research and Quality:

www.ahrq.gov

www.dietaryguidelines.gov

www.health.gov

https://medlineplus.gov

https://www.samhsa.gov

https://www.diabetes.org

www.obesitymedicine.org

www.sleephealth.org

med.upenn.edu/hbhe4

PositivePsychology.com

https://www.uptodate.com

www.cdc.gov

www.fda.gov

www.healthypeople.gov

www.ods.od.nih.gov

www.uspreventiveservicestaskforce.org

www.heart.org

www.sleepfoundation.org

bu.edu/sph

www.niaaa.nih.gov

https://apps.bluezones.com/en/vitality

Other Available Study Tools

Foundations of Lifestyle Medicine Board Review Manual

Lifestyle Medicine: Essential McQs for Certification in Lifestyle Medicine

Brainscape: Search Lifestyle Medicine

Quizlet: Search Lifestyle Medicine, Nutrition

LM Maintenance of Certification

You will likely hear results right around two weeks after the date of the last test. If you pass, you will be able to immediately start appending your title with DipABLM for at least 10 years. You will also receive information on choosing between two recertification options: Lifestyle Medicine Maintenance of Certification (LMMOC) or retest in ten years. The cheapest option seems to be LMMOC. It involves reading three LM articles per year and submitting 30 LM CME every five years. You will receive your physical diploma by the end of January.

CHAPTER TWO
INTRODUCTION TO LIFESTYLE MEDICINE

Lifestyle Medicine is the use of evidence-based lifestyle therapeutic interventions — including whole-food plant-based nutrition, regular physical activity, restorative sleep, stress management, avoidance of harmful substances, and positive social connections — as a primary modality to prevent, treat, and potentially reverse chronic disease. There are several types of methods to help change behavior that are employed, including Intensive Therapeutic Lifestyle Change (ITLC) treatment programs.

Current State of Affairs:
Healthcare spending is approximately 20% of GDP.
Despite high spending, the US consistently ranks low in health system performance regarding outcomes with international comparisons.
Key drivers of rising healthcare costs are pharmaceutical, devices, administrative; followed by higher burden of chronic disease.
The top 10 leading causes of death in the US are almost entirely modifiable by lifestyle choices.

Figure 2-1. Cost Burden of Lifestyle Related Chronic Illness (US)

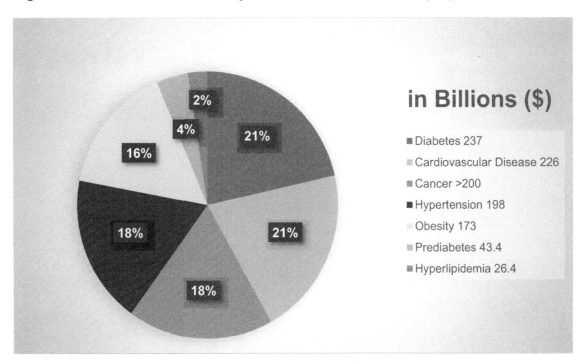

Table 2-1. Lifestyle Medicine Core Competencies

Leadership	Promote healthy behaviors as foundation of medical care
	Practice healthy behavior personally
	Create school/work/home environments that support healthy behavior
Knowledge	Demonstrate knowledge about how specific lifestyle changes can have an impact on patients' health outcomes
	Describe ways physician engagement can have a positive effect on health outcomes
Assessment	Assess social, psychological, and biological predisposition to health behavior
	Assess readiness, willingness, and ability of patient to make a health behavior change
	Perform history and physical relevant to lifestyle medicine and order/interpret appropriate tests
Management Skills	Use nationally recognized practice guidelines
	Establish effective relationships with patients and their families
	Collaborate with patients and their families to develop action plans
	Help patients manage and sustain healthy behavior changes
Office and Community Support	Aim to practice as part of an interdisciplinary team
	Develop and apply office systems and technology
	Measure/report outcomes
	Use appropriate community referral processes

(Source: Lianov and Johnson, Physician Competencies for Prescribing Lifestyle Medicine, JAMA 2010)

Table 2-2. Comparison of Lifestyle Medicine to Other Fields

Field of Medicine	Approach	Modalities
Lifestyle	**Lifestyle behaviors are 1st line and most important (medication and surgery viewed as supplemental).** **The patient takes an active role in their health.**	**Nutrition, physical activity, sleep, emotional health, avoidance of harmful substances, social connection**
Conventional (Western)	Disease focused approach (often infectious, environmental, or genetic)	Medication or surgery is highest level of care
Integrative	Whole-person approach (physical, social, emotional, mental, environmental, and spiritual needs)	Integrates conventional and alternative medical therapies
Functional	Focuses on root cause physiology at the biochemical/cellular level	Investigates cell metabolism, digestive function, detoxification, and control of oxidative stress
Naturopathic	Focuses on natural remedies and addresses whole person (mind, body, spirit)	Herbs, homeopathy, massage, acupuncture, exercise, nutrition, sleep
Alternative / complementary	Methods in place of (alternative) or in addition to (complementary) conventional medicine	Utilized as part of other medical fields
Mindbody	Investigates interaction between body and mind	Relaxation, hypnosis, visual imagery, meditation, yoga, biofeedback, spirituality, tai chi
Preventative	Morbidity and mortality prevention for the public	Emphasizes population-based interventions (screening, vaccination)
Planetary Health	Transdisciplinary social movement-environment degradation, climate change	Carbon footprint reduction via plant-based diet, physical activity as transportation; reduction oxidative stress

Table 2-3. Impact of Health Related Behaviors on Key Health Outcomes

Trial/Study	Methods	Objectives/Outcomes
Nurses' Health Study	Prospective cohort of women (1976): - Phase 1: 121K, OCPs, smoking, cancer, CVD - Phase 2: 116K, OCPs, lifestyle - Phase 3: enrolling	5 risk factors identified (nonsmoker, healthy BMI, physically active, alcohol intake <1 drink/wk, healthy diet) associated with 82% lower risk CAD
Health Professional Follow-up Study	Prospective cohort of 51K men (1985)	Lifestyle and cancer, CVD
Adventist Health Study	Prospective cohort of 7th day Adventists in Loma Linda (1958): - Mortality Study:23K - Phase 1: 34K, cancer and CVD - Phase 2: 96K, diet and cancer	Vegetarian diet associated with reduced rates of all-cause mortality, heart disease, cancer, lower BMI, diabetes, metabolic syndrome Note: Phase 2 included one of the largest cohorts of black Americans to be included in a study
Framingham Heart Study	Prospective cohort 5K (1948)	Identification of CV RF (age, gender, total cholesterol, LDL, SBP, smoking) Greater than two RF associated with increased risk of CVD by 50-60%
National Health and Nutrition Examination Survey (NHANES)	5000 surveys yearly since 1960's, cross sectional analysis	Prediabetes increasing, UPFs increasing Used to report most frequently consumed foods
Chicago Heart Association (CHA) Project	Prospective study 39K (1975)	Favorable CV health (BP, cholesterol, weight, diabetes, smoking) in middle age associated with greater longevity and lower healthcare costs in older age
Women's Health Initiative (WHI)	Prospective study 161K (1991)	Hormone therapy does not prevent heart disease in postmenopausal women; modest increase in hip bone density; no risk reduction for breast/colon cancer
Euro Prospective Investigation into Cancer (EPIC)	Prospective cohort 521K (1993)	Lower meat dietary patterns associated with reduced cancer mortality
Multi-ethnic Study of Atherosclerosis (MESA)	Prospective cohort 6K (2000)	Whole grains, fruits, nuts/seeds, green leafy veggies, low-fat dairy assoc. w 15% red. risk T2DM Strong association between coronary artery calcium scores and CVD
INTERHEART Study	International case control 30K adults with history of MI (2004)	9 RF identified: smoking, elevated ApoB/ApoA1 ratio (lipids), diabetes, hypertension, abdominal obesity (these 5 accounted for 80% of the risk), physical inactivity, diet lacking fruits and vegetables, alcohol, psychosocial factors
INTERSTROKE Study	International case control 27K adults with history of acute stroke (2016)	10 RF identified: smoking, elevated ApoB/ApoA1 ratio (lipids), diabetes, hypertension (primary risk factor for hemorrhagic stroke), abdominal obesity, physical inactivity, diet lacking in fruits and vegetables, alcohol, stress/depression, cardiac causes (responsible for 90% stroke risk)

Table 2-4. Impact of Lifestyle Interventions on Chronic Disease

Trial/Study	Methods	Objectives/Outcomes
Multiple Risk Factor Intervention Trial (MRFIT)	Randomized clinical trial of 12K men (1976)	RF (HTN, HLD, smoking) reduction did not lead to significant changes in CV and total mortality, although results trended toward better outcomes in the intervention group, particularly with longer follow-up
Lyon Diet Heart Study	Randomized controlled trial of 605 adults with history of MI (1995)	Intervention group (Mediterranean diet) had 50-70% lower risk of recurrent heart disease (a secondary prevention study)
Dietary Approaches to Stop Hypertension (DASH)	Randomized controlled trial 459 adults (1993); second study of 412 patients (1997)	DASH (high plants, low fat) diet reduced SBP on average 5 mmHg and DBP on average 3 mmHg within 2 wks; follow-up study correlated low sodium levels with further reductions (SBP by 11 and DBP by 5 mmHg)
Optimal Macronutrient Intake Trial for Heart Health (OmniHeart)	RCT 3 diet types (2003)	Protein and fat predominant diet reduced BP, lipids, CV risk score (but carb rich diet was high in processed refined carbs)
Action to Control Cardiovascular Risk in Diabetes (ACCORD)	Randomized controlled trial of 10K with elevated HbA1c (2008)	Intensive pharmacologic therapy to lower HbA1c *increased mortality* and did not reduce nonfatal events (trial discontinued early)
Complete Health Improvement Program (CHIP)	Randomized clinical trial of 348 adults (2012)	Encouraged plant-based diet and daily physical activity; intervention had greater significant decreases in BMI, weight, and % body fat in patients with diabetes, with a positive return on investment (6-month ROI 2:1)
PREDIMED (**PRE**vencion con **DI**eta **MED**itteranea)	Randomized controlled trial of 7.5K adults at risk for CVD (2013)*	Incidence of major cardiovascular events was lower in group on Mediterranean diet supplemented with olive oil or nuts compared to reduced fat control group (primary prevention study)
Esselstyn Heart Disease Program	Pilot study of 18 patients with severe CAD (1985); follow-up study of 198 patients (2014)	Plant based, very low-fat diet and lipid-lowering medication to reduce cholesterol and secondary CV events
Diabetes Prevention Program	12-month program intensive nutrition and activity intervention for high-risk individuals	T2DM in at-risk adults was reduced by 58% with intensive lifestyle intervention, and by 31% with metformin, compared with placebo

Note: RF = risk factor(s)
*Study was retracted and republished after errors in randomization within households noted, effect estimates were corrected and were similar to original findings.

Table 2-5. Lifestyle Medicine as a High Priority Treatment

Guideline	Chronic Disease
International Society of Hypertension 2020 Global Hypertension Guidelines	Lifestyle medicine "first line" antihypertensive treatment
2019 American College of Cardiology/American Heart Association	Plant based and Mediterranean diets recommended, citing PREDIMED study
American Association of Clinical Endocrinology/American College of Endocrinology	Recommend lifestyle interventions to include nutrition, physical activity, and behavioral modifications
American Academy Pediatrics/Endocrine Society	Intensive lifestyle intervention for high-risk overweight and obese patients (before pharmacotherapy)
American Diabetes Association/Endocrine Society	Lifestyle intervention first line treatment for hyperglycemia in patients over 65yo and a fundamental part of all diabetes care.
American Cancer Society	Cancer prevention recommendations include healthy body weight, nutrition, physical activity and avoidance of alcohol.

Pediatric population also impacted (obesity rates around 20%)-lifestyle interventions effective, especially when parents involved, in reducing cardiovascular risk factors and risks of diabetes mellitus, nonalcoholic fatty liver disease and polycystic ovarian syndrome.

CHAPTER 3
FUNDAMENTALS OF HEALTH BEHAVIOR CHANGE

Definitions

Positive Psychology: The scientific study of what makes life most worth living, focusing on both individual and societal well-being. It studies three pillars-positive subjective experience, positive individual traits, and positive institutions. *(See Chapter 12 for more detail.)*

Self-confidence: The trust a person has in their reasoning, capabilities, and qualities

Self-efficacy: Self-motivation plus self-confidence (the desire and confidence in one's ability to reach a goal); the core of successful health behavior change

Self-motivation: Autonomous or internal motivation; can be increased with coaching

Teachable moment: A time of challenge or transition (acute coronary event or new chronic health diagnosis) that can be an opportunity to encourage lifestyle change, i.e. trigger

Therapeutic Alliance: a measure of the (clinician's) and (patient's) mutual engagement in the work of (treatment)-thus representing an important component for achieving treatment success, regardless of the specific treatment modality employed."

Health Behavior Change Theories

Table 3-1. Health Belief Model

Model	Key Idea	Details/Constructs	Examples
Health Belief Model	Individual beliefs/threat to health	1. Perceived susceptibility 2. Perceived severity 3. Perceived benefit in offered solution 4. Perceived barriers of solution 5. Cues to action 6. Self-efficacy (added later)	Vaccines, early detection, screenings

Figure 3-1. Health Belief Model

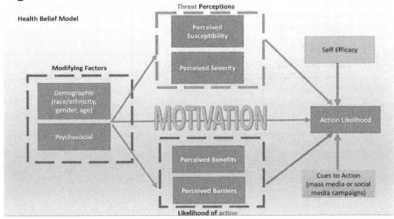

Table 3-2. Theory of Planned Behavior

Model	Key Idea	Details/Constructs	Examples
Theory of Planned Behavior	Behavioral intention - affected by attitude and risk/benefit analysis	1. Attitude 2. Behavioral intention 3. Subjective norms 4. Social norms 5. Perceived power 6. Perceived behavioral control	Advertising, public relations

Figure 3-2. Theory of Planned Behavior

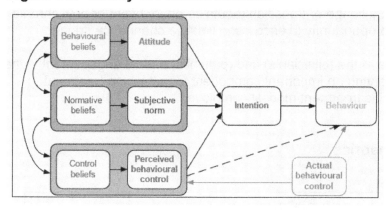

Table 3-3. Social Cognitive Theory

Model	Key Idea	Details/Constructs	Examples
Social Cognitive Theory	Reciprocal interaction of person, environment, and behavior	1. Reciprocal determinism 2. Behavioral capability 3. Observational learning (modeling) 4. Reinforcements 5. Expectations 6. Self-efficacy	Safe sex behavior

Figure 3-3. Social Cognitive Theory

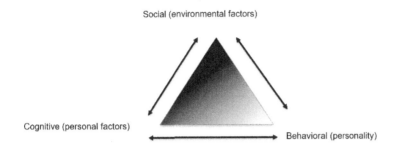

Social (environmental factors)

Cognitive (personal factors)

Behavioral (personality)

Table 3-4. Transtheoretical Model of Change

Model	Key Idea	Details/Constructs	Example
Transtheoretical Model of Change	Stages of change, bidirectional	1. Precontemplation 2. Contemplation 3. Preparation 4. Action 5. Maintenance (6. Termination)	Smoking cessation

Figure 3-4. Transtheoretical Model of Change

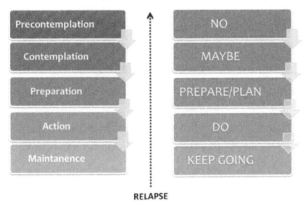

Transtheoretical Model Stages of change

Precontemplation	NO
Contemplation	MAYBE
Preparation	PREPARE/PLAN
Action	DO
Maintanence	KEEP GOING

RELAPSE

Table 3-5. Self-Determination Theory

Model	Key Idea	Details/Constructs	Examples
Self-Determination Theory	Self-motivation and self-determination	1. Autonomy 2. Competence 3. Relatedness	Taking multi-vitamin, healthy eating

Table 3-6. Precaution Adoption Model

Model	Key Idea	Details/Constructs	Example
Precaution Adoption Process	Decision-making based on awareness, unidirectional model	1. Unaware 2. Aware, but unengaged 3. Undecided about acting 4. Desire to act 5. Acting 6. Maintenance	Radon testing

Table 3-7. Diffusion of Innovation Theory

Model	Key Idea	Details/Constructs	Examples
Diffusion of Innovation Theory	How an idea gains momentum	1. Innovators 2. Early adopters 3. Early majority 4. Late majority 5. Laggards	New forms of birth control, technology

Table 3-8. Organization Development Theory

Model	Key Idea	Details/Constructs	Example
Organizational Development Theory	Organizational structures and processes influence worker behavior and motivation	1. Organizational climate 2. Organizational culture 3. Diagnosis 4. Action planning 5. Intervention 6. Evaluation	Improving clinical efficiency and flow

14

Table 3-9. Organizational Behavior Model

Model	Key Idea	Details/Constructs	Examples
Organizational Behavior Model	How people behave in organizational work environments motivation	Micro: individuals (intra/interpersonal) Meso: groups/ communities Macro: organizations/ systems	Micro: motivation, attitude, emotions Meso: team dynamics, leadership Macro: organization design, climate

Figure 3-5. Ecological Systems Theory (Bronfenbrenner)

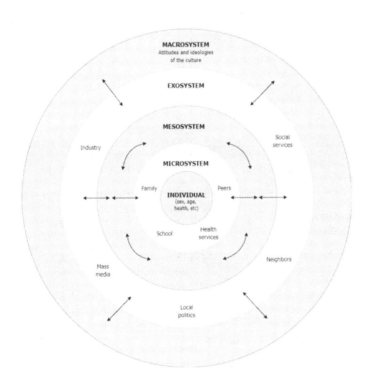

Table 3-10. Social Determinants of Health

Economic Stability	Neighborhood and Physical Environment	Education	Food	Community and Social Context	Healthcare System
Income	Housing	Literacy	Food desert	Safety	Insurance coverage
Debt	Utilities	Language barrier	Insecurity	Gender Inequality	Provider availability
Employment	Crime rates	Early childhood education		Racial Segregation	Culture/language barrier
Medical bills	Transportation			Domestic violence	Access
	Parks/walkability			Adverse Childhood Experiences (ACE)	

Table 3-11. Patient-Provider Strategies for Stages of Change

Readiness level	Confidence level	Status / time frame	Patient comment	Possible response	Discussion	Coaching technique
Pre-contemplation	0-3	No change in foreseeable future	"I don't/can't need/want to change"	"How will you know when it's time to change?"	Health risks associated with specific behavior and benefits of change	MI, PP
Contemplation	4-6	Considering change within 6 months	"I've thought about it"	"Are you considering a change in the next month?"	Personalize health risks; pros and cons of change	MI, PP
Preparation	7*	Planning change within next month or action recently taken	"I am ready to make a change"	Co-create action plan, assess confidence levels	Possible barriers, enhancing commitment level	CBT, PP
Action	8-9	Change started- inconsistent or may not have met goals, <6months	"I am changing"	"What is giving you the most trouble?" "How can your support network help you?"	Modify action plan, review barriers that come up, social support system	CBT, PP
Maintenance	10	Goal reached and remained consistent for >6 months	"I have changed"	"You are doing well." "What obstacles have you ovecome and how?"	Coping strategies for stress reduction, problem-solving	CBT, PP
Termination		No longer thinking of it as a change	"I have no desire to return to my old habit"			

*If the patient's score is above 7, patient is more likely to accomplish her/his goal.
(Notes: MI = motivational interviewing   PP = positive psychology   CBT = cognitive behavioral therapy)

Table 3-12. Steps in Creating a Lifestyle Medicine Action Plan

	Step	Example
1	Explain your role as provider	Expert (medical diagnosis/risks) and coach (collaborate on action plan)
2	Share diagnosis and potential risks of inaction	HTN/risks of acute coronary events
3	Describe evidence-based lifestyle medicine prescriptions	Incorporate 150 min per week of moderate exercise
4	Recognize progress made	Patient has been walking twice a week with a friend; use positive psychology to affirm and encourage
5	Determine area for change	Brisk walk 3-4 days a week; collaborate with patient
6	Assess patient's confidence and importance levels	On a scale of 1-10, how confident are you (how important is it to you) that you be able to master this change in the next 3-6 months?
7	If score is >7, ask patient to elaborate on her/his goals	If not, inquire as to why the score is low and what she/he could do to increase confidence; or choose new area.
8	Follow **SMART** goal format when writing action plan: • **S**pecific • **M**easurable • **A**ttainable • **R**elevant • **T**imebound	I will walk on my treadmill at a speed where I can speak (but not sing) at a 3% incline for 30 min twice a week before work I will continue to walk twice a week with my friend at a similar pace. I will commit to doing this for the next four weeks.

Table 3-12 (cont.). Steps in Creating a Lifestyle Medicine Action Plan

	Step	Example
9	Ask patient about anything she/he needs to achieve goal	Resources, support systems
10	Create strategies to overcome identified obstacles/barriers	What if it's raining/my friend cancels?
11	Connect patient with support systems	Family members, local support groups, group coaching and shared medical appointments, online, tech
12	Confirm patient's commitment	Patient to sign, date, and keep a copy; copy in chart
13	Implement accountability	Self-monitoring systems/apps
14	Schedule follow up (in person, virtual, or telephone)	Follow-up in one month

Table 3-13. The Five A's of Health Behavior Change

Assess	Identify health risks, readiness	
Advise	Explain how changing behavior can impact future health	Lifestyle Prescription
Agree	Focus change and collaborate on specific goals	Action Plan (SMART)
Assist	Address barriers, relapse prevention planning, provide resources	
Arrange	Follow-up/support	Referrals

For alcohol evaluation the steps are: Ask, Advise, Assess, Assist, Arrange (see Chapter 10)

Table 3-14. Ways to Build Therapeutic Alliance

Coaching: The process of empowering someone to develop the knowledge, skills, resources, and confidence to enact and sustain changes

Therapeutic alliance is built on trust (Trust is the willingness to be vulnerable based on benevolence, honesty, openness, reliability, competence)

Coaching Role			
Environment	Treatment	Follow-Up	Patient Tools for Self-Management
Use inclusive language (we, us)	Offer an intervention	Reiterate coaching role	CBT *(see Table 3-17)*
Use people-first language (a person "with diabetes" instead of "a diabetic")	Match intervention to readiness level	Review/update diagnoses and action plans from last visit	Social support, community, employee programs
Ask permission around sensitive subjects (assessing weight, alcohol use)	Empower patient by encouraging her/his own ideas	Utilize positive psychology to affirm patient's progress and highlight her/his strengths	Digital technology (wearables, telehealth, tracking apps)
Acknowledge previous efforts in a positive way	Discuss support network with patient (family, friends, support groups, peer programs)	If goals unmet, make revisions based on confidence level If previous goals met, congratulate, and inquire as to which goal patient is ready to master next	Behavior contracts (evidence inconclusive): - "aids" - not real contracts - clarifies goals - developing the contract can be therapeutic in itself - accountability
Inspire awareness	Create an action plan *(see Table 3-12)*	Create new action plan(s)	"Skill power" over willpower: - Put together an algorithm to encourage long-term success *("When I feel X, I will do Y instead of Z")*
	Collaborate with qualified health and wellness coaches in your area*	Review progress made/summarize future directions	

(*Source: National Board Health & Wellness Coaching (NBHWC) directory)

Benefits of Positive Psychology

- Improve attention, open-mindedness, creativity, and ability to reach a strategic perspective
- Builds resilience, reinforces autonomy and self-efficacy
- Vital for brain learning in-the-moment and successful behavior change over time
- Emphasizes current strengths, skills, and abilities
- Increases therapeutic alliance between provider and patient

Table 3-15. Motivational Interviewing

Fundamentals (RECS)	
Roll with resistance	Remain non-judgmental, listen, encourage patient to continue to share, let patient talk but may need to redirect to a new area where more change talk can be explored
Empathy	Show understanding and share patient's feelings; empathy fuels collaboration
Contrast between present and goal	Show the difference between where patient is and where she/he wants to be, allow patient to form conclusions
Support self-efficacy	Build patient confidence in her/his ability to succeed
Core Skills (OARS)	
Open ended questions	"What", "How", "Tell me more"; encourage a narrative; explore experiences, expectations, needs, feelings, priorities
Affirmations	Use "you" pronoun, recognize patient's strengths, efforts
Reflections *(see Table 3-16)*	Repeat the statement back to patient to show understanding, interest, empathy, and to bring awareness
Summarize	Use as transition between topics or at end of visit
5 R's	
Relevance	Consequences specific to patient
Risks	Acute/long term effects on self/others
Rewards of behavior change	Benefits to health, financial, social/family
Roadblocks	Social, perceived withdrawal, fear of failure
Repetition	Multiple methods/attempts

Table 3-16. Types of Reflections in Motivational Interviewing

	Description	Patient	Provider
Simple	Paraphrase without added emphasis	"I know I need to change things, but I don't know where to start."	"You can't decide."
Complex	A more powerful choice of words when paraphrasing	"I know I need to change things, but I don't know where to start."	"You may be feeling overwhelmed and are finding it hard to set goals."
Amplified	Accurate, direct, but more exaggerated; used to evoke an "argument" from the patient in favor of change	"I am here because my husband says I drink too much."	"Your alcohol use is completely healthy and you have absolutely no concerns about it."
Double-sided	Show two simultaneous perspectives (readiness and resistance)	"I know I need to exercise more, but I just don't have time."	"You are aware that exercising would be a benefit to you AND you realize that your schedule is busy."
Redirection	Shift focus from area of resistance to a new area	"I have tried all kinds of diets and never had success. I am so sick of dieting."	"You have put a lot of energy into your eating habits, let's explore another area such as physical activity."
Reframing	Invite to see things from another perspective	"Every time I try to stop smoking, I fail."	"You have had the courage and determination to try in the past, and tobacco dependence is a chronic illness with relapses being very common."
Elicitation	Elicit-Provide-Elicit (Ask, Listen, Inform) Respects patient autonomy and knowledge base; avoids retelling	"I know that already"	"Tell me what you know about the risk of ultra processed foods to your health"

Table 3-17. Cognitive Behavioral Therapy (CBT) Basics

Provider preparation (things to do before you walk into the room)	1. Discover your internal dialogue (e.g. biases, etc.) 2. Identify which cognitive distortions are present 3. Write factual statements to replace distortions 4. Practice
Recognize nonproductive thinking	Cognitive distortions *(see Table 3-19)*
Explore	Assist the patient to become more aware of her/his thoughts, emotions, and resulting behaviors May use MI reflection skills
Reframe	Help the patient see the situation differently, substitute a more realistic interpretation, foster a new self-talk
Expose	Underlying beliefs that can interfere

Table 3-18. ABCDE's of Cognitive Behavioral Therapy

A	What ACTION or event occurred?	What happened?
B	What BELIEFS do you have about what happened?	What do you think about it?
C	What are the CONSEQUENCES of those beliefs/how do they make you feel?	How does that make you feel?
D	How can you DISPUTE those beliefs?	What's another way to think about it?
E	What EFFECT does the new thoughts process have on how you feel?	How do I feel now?

Table 3-19. Ten Common Cognitive Distortions and Reframed Thoughts

	Definition	Example	Reframed
All-or-nothing	No in-between	"I haven't done anything good in my life since college."	"The fact that I finished college is something to be proud of."
Overgeneralization	Limited factual evidence to support a firm belief	"My husband never does anything nice for me."	"Although it may not be as often as I'd like, I appreciate the times my husband has gone out of his way to make me feel special."
Mental filter	Singling out one bad aspect of a situation	"I got scolded during my annual work review."	"I see now there are areas of growth I can focus, but I am proud of the areas I did well in."
Mind reading	Knowing what another is thinking without asking	"I know my husband thinks I'm a slob."	"I wonder if my husband would like to talk about what his expectations for me are around the house."
Fortune telling	Knowing what will happen as a result of a choice made now	"If I try to change my nutrition habits, my family won't eat it."	"I should include my family in looking for new recipes we might all enjoy."
Magnification/ minimization	Emphasize the minor things and minimize the major things	"I can only lift 5 lb. dumbbells at the gym."	"I am proud that I have been going to the gym regularly and look forward to building up my strength."
Personalization/ blame	You/another completely responsible for the blame	"That customer was a jerk and so rude. She or He really ruined my day."	"That customer may be struggling to pay bills or just lost a loved one; they likely weren't trying to make me mad on purpose."
Emotional reasoning	Feelings don't lie	"I feel like a failure."	"I feel awful today, but everyone has bad days and tomorrow is a new day."

Table 3-19 (cont.). Ten Common Cognitive Distortions and Reframed Thoughts

	Definition	Example	Reframed
(Mis)labeling	Defining oneself with an unhelpful term	"I am so annoying; I talk way too much."	"I am extroverted and enjoy talking to others."
Disqualifying the positive	Acknowledging the good but assigning it no value	"Cutting back on alcohol will help me sleep better, but then I can't hang out with my friends."	"Reducing alcohol may be hard around my friends, but I can find non-alcoholic drinks to enjoy and the benefit to my sleep and overall health will be worth it."

Figure 3-6. Relapse Prevention Planning

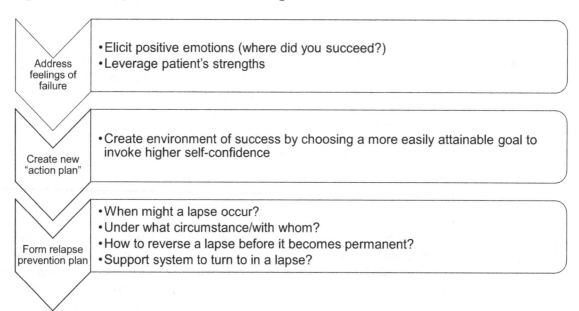

Address feelings of failure
- Elicit positive emotions (where did you succeed?)
- Leverage patient's strengths

Create new "action plan"
- Create environment of success by choosing a more easily attainable goal to invoke higher self-confidence

Form relapse prevention plan
- When might a lapse occur?
- Under what circumstance/with whom?
- How to reverse a lapse before it becomes permanent?
- Support system to turn to in a lapse?

Table 3-20. Supporting Studies

Methods	Question/Intervention	Takeaway
Physicians' Use of the 5As in counseling obese patients: Is the quality of counseling associated with patients' motivation and intention to lose weight? *BMC Health Serv Res* (2010)		
Cross-sectional (N=137)	Does the quality of 5As counseling affect patient motivation/intention?	Assess and Advise used the most; Agree, Assist and Arrange much less. The more counseling techniques used, the higher the motivation and intention scores.
Effect on health-related outcomes of interventions to alter the interaction. Between patients and practitioners: a systematic review of trials. *Ann Fam Med* (2004)		
Systematic review of RCTs (35 studies)	*Intervention examples:* - *Helping patient take a more active role (elicit questions/concerns)* - *Enhance provider approach (pay attention more to emotions, match coaching to patient's personality, providing more info)*	*Outcomes positively affected in about 40% of studies.* *Complexity not necessary for impact.* *Evidence lacking given lack of standardized interventions, theoretical underpinning, and objective outcomes.*
Physicians' empathy and clinical outcomes for diabetic patients. *Acad Med* (2011)		
Cross-sectional (N=891)	HbA1C, LDL-C, provider empathy scores	Providers with higher empathy scores from patients achieved better HbA1C control (56% vs 40%) and LDL-C control (59% vs 44%)
Physician Communication Techniques and Weight Loss in Adults *Am J Prev Med* (2010)		
Cohort (N=461)	Motivational interviewing (MI) techniques while discussing weight loss	Counseling with MI trained provider led to 1.6kg weight loss, counseling with untrained provides led to maintenance or weight gain

(Note: RCT = Randomized Controlled Trial)

Table 3-21. Patient Resource Guide

Nutrition	1. ACLM's Six Pillars: Nutrition Handout Academy of Nutrition and Dietetics 2. Online and mobile nutrition trackers 3. Medically tailored meals 4. Meal preparation or delivery services 5. Governmental food assistance programs 6. Healthy People 2030
Physical Activity	1. ACLM's Six Pillars: Activity Handout 2. The American College of Sports Medicine Exercise is Medicine resources 3. Center for Disease Control and Prevention (CDC) Physical Activity Guidelines
Sleep	1. ACLM's Six Pillars: Sleep Handout 2. American Academy of Sleep Medicine 3. Online and mobile sleep trackers and wearables
Social Relationships	1. ACLM's Six Pillars: Social Relationships Handout 2. Local and community-based organization engagement and volunteering
Stress	1. ACLM's Six Pillars: Stress Handout 2. Online and mobile programs and applications
Avoiding Risky Substance Use	1. ACLM's Six Pillars: Avoiding Risky Substances Handout 2. CDC Alcohol Resources 3. Smokefree.gov

CHAPTER 4
KEY CLINICAL PROCESSES IN LIFESTYLE MEDICINE

This chapter summarizes the key clinical processes of a lifestyle medicine practice. You can directly apply the contents of this chapter to your clinical work in addition to the exam.

Table 4-1. Components of LM Vital Signs

Vital Sign	Units	Scoring	Other
Temperature	F or C	95 – 100.4	
Heart Rate	Beats per minute	60 – 90	
Blood Pressure**	mmHg	See Table 4-3	Confirm with non-clinic BP reading
Respiratory Rate	Breaths per minute	8 – 18	
Pulse O2	SpO2	>95	Or as per baseline
Body Mass Index**	kg/m^2 or lbs/in^2	See Table 4-4	Controversial
Diet	Servings/day of vegetables, fruits, whole grains, nuts/seeds, legumes, spices, low-fat dairy, sugar-sweetened beverages, packaged foods, fried foods, high-fat dairy, meat, eggs	See Table 4-9 for options	May use team-member to gather data
Physical Activity	Physical Activity Vital Sign*: Days/week; min/day		Assess strength separately (d/wk)
Emotional Well-being	In most ways, life close to ideal; satisfied w/ life	1-5, where 5=high	Low scores were associated w/ race
Stress	Perceived Stress Score	Use PSS rubric	
Sleep	Typical weekday hrs, typical weekend hrs, perceived quality	See Chapter 9	Epworth Sleepiness Scale
Tobacco use	Packs/year equivalent for each form of tobacco	See Chapter 10	+ second-hand exposure
Alcohol consumption	Audit 1Q, if failed then 3Q (Audit-C), if failed then 10Q	See Chapter 10	Once per year

*PAVS is the only validated vital sign.
**Medicare Annual Wellness Visits require measuring of BP and BMI (or waist circumference).

Table 4-2. Clinical Steps to a Lifestyle Medicine (LM) Encounter

Step 1	Ask patient to fill out pre-visit questionnaire(s) regarding medical history, current lifestyle, and disease-specific screening tools prior to your visit	See Table 4-9 through 4-10
Step 2	Review answers to pre-visit questions, take a thorough history, check vital signs, do a physical, and review results	See Tables 4-3 through 4-8
Step 3	Make diagnosis and recommendations	See Chapters 6-11
Step 4	Assess readiness and make action plan	See Chapter 3
Step 5	Coordinate multi-disciplinary care, referrals, and testing as needed	See Tables 4-11 through 4-13

Table 4-3. Blood Pressure

Classification	Systolic Range*	Diastolic Range	MAP
Hypotension			<65
Normal	≤120	≤80	≥65
Elevated	121-129	≤80	
Stage 1	130-139	81-89	
Stage 2	≥140	≥90	

Normal variant to have slightly higher SBP in one arm consistently, usually R>L.

Hypertension (HTN)
-   Prevalence increases with age. 74.5% of people over 60 years have HTN.
-   Diagnosis requires at least two readings over two separate visits.
-   It's also a good idea to get a reading in a non-clinic setting.

Table 4-4. Body Mass Index Cutoffs

BMI = weight/height^2 * 703 in U.S. (lbs and in)
BMI = weight/height^2 everywhere else (kg and m)

Classification	Non-Asian	Asian-Pacific**
Underweight	<18.5	<18.5
Normal	18.5-24.9	18.5-22.9
Overweight	25-29.9	22.9-25
Pre-Obesity*		25-29.9
Obesity, Class I	30-34.9	30-34.9
Obesity, Class II	35-39.9	35-39.9
Obesity, Class III	≥40	≥40

Treat the same as obesity, Class I
**It was determined that Asians (Chinese, Japanese, Korean, and South Asians) are at higher risk of diabetes at lower BMI cutoffs.*

Table 4-5. Waist Circumference and Waist/Hip Ratio Cutoffs

	Female	Male
Waist Circumference	<35 inches	<40 inches
Waist/Hip Ratio	≤0.85	≤0.9

Physical activity and body composition assessments – See Chapter 8

Table 4-6. Screening and Diagnostic Laboratory Tests

Name of Test	Notes
CBC	If anemic, iron studies
CMP	Kidney, liver, electrolytes
Fasting lipids	See Table 4-8
>>>LDL breakdown	More detailed cholesterol analysis
Fasting serum glucose, HbA1c, OGTT	See Table 4-7
Fasting serum insulin, C-peptide, HOMA-IR	More detailed diabetes screening
Vitamin D	
TSH, total/free T4	

Table 4-7. Diabetes Diagnosis*

	Normal	Pre-DM	DM	Partial Remission	Complete Remission	Prolonged Remission
Fasting Blood Glucose	<100	100-124	≥125	100-125	<100	<100
HbA1c	<5.7	5.7-6.4	≥6.5	<6.5	<5.7	<5.7
2-Hour Oral Glucose Tolerance Test (OGTT) (75g)	<140	140-199	≥200			
TIME			Requires repeat testing, unless unequivocal	≥1 year	≥1 year	≥5 year
THERAPY				No active pharmaceuticals or surgery		

*Begin screening at age 35 if overweight or obese. Other risk factors include:
- Pre-diabetes
- History of CVD
- HTN with BP ≥140/90 or on HTN meds
- Signs of insulin resistance
- High risk race (Asian or Pacific Islander, Black, Hispanic, Native American)
- Physical inactivity
- First degree relative w/ T2DM
- Women with PCOS, delivered a baby >9 lbs, or had gestational DM

Table 4-8. Cholesterol Cutoffs

Lipid	American Normal	Ideal LM Range	Notes
Total Cholesterol (TC)	<200	90-140 (2.327-3.62 mmol/L)*	If <150 mg/dL, stops plaque progress
HDL	>40	>50	
LDL=TC-HDL-(TG*0.2)	<100	≤70 (1.81 mmol/L)	If TG>400, invalid calculation
Triglycerides (TG)	<200	<150	
High-sensitivity C-reactive protein			
Apolipoprotein B	<130	≥130	Better than LDL-C
Lp(a)	<50	≥50	>1.5 inc risk of CVD

Table 4-9. LM Pillar-Specific Questionnaires

LM Pillar	Questionnaires	More Info
Diet and Nutrition	Numerous, 3-day food diary, photograph meals, NIH dietary assessments, Starting the Conversation (8 items), Mediterranean Diet Adherence Screener (MEDAS), Automated Self-administered 24-Hour Dietary Assessment Tool, Dietary History Questionnaire	Sometimes requires pre-education (e.g. teach portion size before 3-day food diary)
Physical Activity	PAVS + strength, International Physical Activity Questionnaire (IPAQ), Physical Activity Readiness Questionnaire for Everyone (PAR-Q+)	Also ask about daily sedentary behavior
Emotional and Mental Well-Being	Satisfaction with Life Scale (SWLS), Perceived Stress Scale Assessment, Patient Health Questionnaire (PHQ) Tools, General Anxiety Disorder (GAD) Tools, Beck Depression/Anxiety Inventory, Diagnostic and Statistical Manual (DSM-5) depression and anxiety criteria questions	Chapter 8
Sleep	Single-Item Sleep Quality Scale, Global Sleep Assessment Questinnaire, STOP-BANG, Epworth Sleepiness Scale (ESS), Pittsburgh Sleep Quality Index (PSQI)	Chapter 9
Toxic Substances	National Inst on Drug Abuse; Tobacco, Alcohol, Prescription Meds, and other Substances; CAGE, Alcohol Use Disorder Identification Test (AUDIT_C);	Chapter 10
Social Connectedness / Positive Psychology	Loma Linda social Relationship questionnaire, A Brief Model of Social support, Social Support for diet/exercise, VIA Character Survey	Chapter 11

Table 4-10. Other Questionnaires, Including Disease-Specific Screening Tools

Name	Purpose	Special Notes
Lifestyle Assessment Short (2 pages) / Long (14 pages) Form	Assess all lifestyle factors	ACLM + Loma Linda; English and Spanish; not validated
Life's Simple 7 Questionnaire (smoking, physical activity, weight, diet, fasting glucose, cholesterol, and BP)	Cardiovascular disease	American Heart Association; if 5/7 good, then 78% reduction in CV death
Atherosclerotic Cardiovascular Disease (ASCVD) Risk Estimator Plus (age, gender, TC, HDL, LDL, smoking, DM, HTN meds, use of statin or aspirin)	Risk of MI in next 10 yrs in adults 20-79 years old w/o heart disease; low, borderline, intermediate, or high	American College of Cardiology; non-Hispanic white and black adults; underestimates for Native Americans, south Asians, and Puerto Ricans; overestimates for East Asians and Mexican Americans
Multi-Ethnic Study of Atherosclerosis (MESA) risk score	10-year coronary heart disease risk in men and women	Validated, includes coronary calcium score; 2015
Reynold's risk score	CVD in women	Includes family history and high sensitivity CRP
Prediabetes Risk Test	Diabetes	Center for Disease Control (CDC)
Diabetes Risk Test	Diabetes	American Diabetes Association (ADA)
Framingham Risk Score for Hard Coronary Heart Disease	10-year risk of MI	Non-diabetic, ages 30-79, no prior history of cardiac disease or intermittent claudication
Finnish Diabetes Risk Score (FINDRISC)	Diabetes within 10 years	Finnish Diabetes Association
Australian T2DM Risk (AUSDRISK)	Diabetes	Australian government
12- or 36-Item Short Form (SF-12 or SF 36)	Overall well-being	RAND Corporation
Electronic Preventive Services Selector (ePSS)	Screening, counseling, and preventive services	Agency for Healthcare Research Quality indicators (AHRQ); from Prescription for Health initiative
Healthy Body Calculator	Customized nutrition / physical activity recommendation	Ask the Dietician
Harris-Benedict Equation Calculator	Basal Energy Expenditure	CDC

Table 4-11. LM Guidelines for Chronic Diseases

Cardiovascular Disease, Hyperlipidemia, and Hypertension
Cardiovascular Disease
Calorie neutral or negative
150 min moderate physical activity or 75 min vigorous physical activity per week
Emphasize fruits, vegetables, whole grains, plant-based proteins, legumes, nuts, fish, and low-fat/nonfat dairy. For meat, eat lean and unprocessed.
Eat high fiber foods
No tobacco use, stay within alcohol use guidelines (see Chapter 10)
Limit salt and sugar
Statin for $\geq$ 1 RF, age 40-75, and ASCVD $\geq$ 10%
ACLM: low-fat, whole foods plant-based diet to reduce plaque build up
Hyperlipidemia
Same as CVD, and limit saturated fat to less than 6% of daily calories
Eliminate or severely limit red meat, dairy, and fried foods
Hypertension
DASH diet with Sodium < 2,300mg/day or < 1,500mg/day (see Tables 2-4 & 6-17)
No tobacco use, stay within alcohol use guidelines (see Chapter 10)

Diabetes
150 min moderate physical activity or 75 min vigorous physical activity per week
Diabetes Plate: Fill half plate with non-starchy vegetables, ¼ with whole grains/starchy vegetables, and ¼ with lean proteins, like beans. Drink water or calorie-free beverages, only.
Avoid ultra-processed foods, trans fats, sugary drinks, and alcohol.
No tobacco use
Eliminate added sugar
ACLM: low-fat, whole foods, lower calorie, plant-based diet to induce DM remission
Consider intensive programs when available

Weight Loss
Reduce calories by 3,500/week → -1 lb/week; F: 1,200-1,500 calories/day; M: 1,500-1,800 calories/day
Increase energy expenditure in conjunction with calorie reduction 500 calories expenditure/day (walking 5 miles/day) → -1 lb/week
Bariatric surgery for BMI ≥ 40, BMI ≥ 35 + obesity comorbidity, BMI ≥ 30 with DM
For CVD patients, weight loss <2-5% improves glucose, HbA1c, triglycerides, systolic BP and >5% improves diastolic BP, HDL, and dec meds
Risk factors for obesity: energy homeostasis, hormonal regulation, genetic predisposition, developmental exposures, the microbiome, environmental or social influences, toxins, and endocrine-disrupting chemicals
Plateau phenomenon – Can last several months to years. Energy expenditure decreases because of leaner and more efficient muscles. Brain and metabolism must also adapt.

Cancer
Healthy weight
150-300 min of mod-vig activity/week. Near 300 min is ideal. Limit sedentary behavior.
Emphasize whole grains, variety of vegetables and fruits, and beans
Limit ultra-processed foods, red and processed meat, sugar-sweetened beverages, refined grains, alcohol, cancer prevention supplements,
Breast feed when possible to reduce own breast cancer risk
Follow standard of care for any cancer therapy recs
Safe sex, get vaccines against Hep B and HPV
Adequate UV sun protection
Avoid urban air pollution, tobacco
Regular cancer screenings, including Hep C, mammogram, CA-125, pap smears, PSA, and colonoscopy/cologuard

33

Table 4-12. Evidence for LM Therapy

Trial	Summary
Lifestyle Heart Trial (5y RCT)	Sustainability of intensive lifestyle changes and effects on CHD compared to statins with better results in lifestyle group
Percutaneous coronary angioplasty compared w/ exercise training in stable CAD	Both groups improved significantly, but significant cost-saving with exercise group
DiRECT (12m RCT)	Intensive weight management vs. standard of care for remission of DM. Weight loss more effective in intensive group and remission was associated with weight loss.
Diabetes Prevention Program, DPP (~2.8y RCT)	Prevent DM with lifestyle vs. metformin. Lifestyle and metformin both helped, but lifestyle was more effective.
Dietary portfolio of chol-lowering foods v.s statin on lipids and CRP (3m RCT)	Low sat fat diet that added plant sterols, viscous fibers, soy protein, and nuts vs. statins in reducing cholesterol. Statin and dietary portfolio were the same.
Comparative effectiveness of exercise and drug interventions on mortality	Exercise vs. drug interventions on mortality. Exercise better in stroke, same in CHD, prediabetes, and worse in CHF than diuretics.
Intensive lifestyle therapy for reversal newly dx'ed DMII in young Asian Indian adults	Low calorie and brisk walking diet for 2 years. High rates of reversal in young adults.
Exercise for depression (meta-analysis)	Exercise is moderately more effective than controls for reducing symptoms of depression, but not more effective than pharmacologic or psychologic therapies.
Therapeutic lifestyle change intervention for improved metabolic syndrome +/- amlodipine/atorvastatin (12m RCT)	Patients with metabolic syndrome were either lifestyle intervention + placebo or lifestyle intervention + amlodipine/atorvastatin. They were comparable. Weight change positively correlated with improvement in metabolic syndrome.

Table 4-13. Resources Lists to Maintain

Resource Type	What to Maintain
Community-based (e.g. Diabetes Prevention Program)	Contact info, eligibility requirements, cost, and if insurance accepted
Clinicians (referrals)	Specialists and ancillary service providers whose practices align with LM
Coaching	Virtual or in-person, cost/ins, program details
Media	Social media accounts to follow or groups to join, handouts on specific topics, documentaries or movies
	National Diabetes Education Program National Diabetes Prevention Program Smokers' Helpline American Heart Association - Getting Healthy tab Million Hearts Initiative 211 Agency on Aging

Table 4-14. Team Members and Roles in LM Practice

Team Member(s)	Role
Administration / Front-desk staff	Check in/check out, billing, scheduling, coordination of referrals
Medical Assistant or Nurse	Vital signs, pre-visit assessments
Physician	Clinical encounter
Health Coach (or any clinician on the team)	Health coaching, can be weekly
Registered Dietician / Nutritionist	Assist with food choices
Physical / Occupational Therapist	Musculoskeletal therapy
Exercise Physiologist / Fitness Trainer	Custom Exercise Programs
Pharmacist	Oversee med regimens and de-escalation
Health Educators	Assist with group visits
Psychologist	Behavioral therapy, cognitive roadblocks
LM Specialists (e.g. ITLC)	More rapid changes
Chiropractor, massage therapist, acupuncturist	Integrative health providers

Ensure lists are in line with Lifestyle Medicine.

Table 4-15. Ten Characteristics of an Interdisciplinary Team

Positive leadership and management	Communication strategies and structures	Personal rewards, training, and development	Appropriate resources and procedures	Appropriate mix of skills
Supportive team climate	Individuals with supportive team-building characteristics	Clear vision	Quality outcomes	Respect and understanding of roles

Nancarrow, S. et al. Ten principles of good interdisciplinary teamwork. Hum Resour Health. 2013 May 10; 11:19.

Table 4-16. Tracking Patients Electronically

Metrics to Track	Where to Track	How Frequently to Track/Notes
Vital signs	Patient Notes	Each visit, at least monthly
Answers to scored screening tools	Patient Notes	On initial visit and annually
Lab results	Patient Notes, EHR reports	On initial, then 3rd, 6th, 12th months of active changes, and then annually
Pre-diabetes or diabetes diagnosis	EHR reports	As per community needs assessment (consider annually)
Pre-hypertension or hypertension diagnosis	EHR reports	As per community needs assessment (consider annually)
Multiple reportable metrics	HEDIS	Annually, uses CPT II codes
Patient Activation Measure	Patient reported	Evals patient engagement in their health
Therapeutic alliance	Many scales	Freudian idea; evals patient-provider relationship

Table 4-17. Group Visits / Shared Medical Appointments (SMAs) / Drop-In Group Medical Appointments (DIGMAs)

What is it?	Approximately 8-12 patients who could benefit from similar education for 90-120 minutes appointment, including some education, discussion, and 1-on-1 visit
Are there variations on this format?	The format is extremely flexible. Many variations exist, including virtual or in-person or combination, series or one-off, home-made lectures or licensed content, no or limited 1-on-1 visits
How many providers are required?	At least one 1 MD/DO/NP, and typically a second individual (to continue discussion if 1-on-1 visits ongoing) (ACLM says 2-4)
Does Medicare cover this?	It is billed as individual visits as long as basic elements of a visit are met and documented
What about confidentiality?	Patients sign a waiver of HIPAA for any information they choose to disclose in a group setting
Why choose this?	Preferred format for many physicians and patients; improved outcomes, though there is a self-selection bias; elements of group therapy and support groups are inherent; saves time; costs less

Table 4-18. Useful LM EHR and Apps (not on exam)

App	Purpose	Other Notes
Pro-Patient Tech	LM EHR with built-in action items, resources, and AI note features	New platform, free trial, then $
MyFitnessPal	Highly integrated food diary	iOS, Android; free for calories or $ for macro/micronutrient content
Cronomoter	Food/exercise diary w/ micronutrient data	iOS, Android; free for patients, $ for professional version
MyPlate Calorie Counter	Food diary, offers food plans for special diets	From Livestrong; iOS, Android; free for calories or $ for macro/micronutrient content
CalorieKing	Reference app for macronutrient data, including fast food	iOS, Android; free w ads
ControlMyWeight	Food diary	From CalorieKing; iOS or website; free
LoseIt	Diet and exercise diary	iOS, Android; free or $ for integration, food plan, etc.
Noom	Coaching, food diary	iOS, Android; $
Healthwatch 360		
Caspia	Health note-taking, symptom tracking	iOS; free
FitBit	Exercise and biometric tracking	iOS, android; equipment cost
Smartwatch	Biometric tracking	iOS, android; Equipment cost
MapMyRun	Exercise tracking	
Finch	Self-care exercises	iOS, android; free or $ for more exercises

Table 4-19. Collaborative and Chronic Care Models

What is it?	Multi-disciplinary team approach to patient care, with the use of pre-determined, collaborating, synergistic team of health professionals
Are there variations on this format?	The format is extremely flexible. The only commonality is that the physician is not the patient's only caregiver.
What are the other different health professionals involved?	Options from Ornish Spectrum Program include: registered dietician, chef/food services, registered nurse, exercise physiologist, health coach, stress management specialist, group support specialist, admin/medical assistant, and marketing director
Does Medicare cover this?	Certain programs have received government funding; also, value-based incentive care is another way to access funds
Which patients is this ideal for?	For patients who need extra support and medical supervision in their lifestyle change; for more motivated / engaged patients who are willing to make changes at a faster pace
Why choose this?	Better, more sustained outcomes than either physician or dietician alone, provides support for the physicians, gives each health professional a valuable role in patient care
Examples of programs	Ornish Spectrum Program Medical fitness collaboration VA's Whole Health Model Diabetes Prevention Program (health coach) Model: Collaborative Care Manager Model (AHRQ) Model: Value-based care Model: The Chronic Care Model (MacColl Institute)

Evidence for FFS primary care and office-based models for lifestyle modification comes from Prescription for Health:
- Six-year initiative funded by Robert Wood Johnson Foundation and AHRQ
- Funded 22 primary care practices to create 27 different strategies
- Purpose: Improve delivery and effectiveness of health behavior change services targeting tobacco use, risky alcohol use, unhealthy diet, and physical inactivity
- All are evidence-based

Outside of FFS, other types of models for primary care include Direct Primary Care and Concierge medicine, in which subscription type payment models are more aligned with the needs of LM care.

Other places to access LM care include specialty clinics, such as obesity medicine, diabetes clinics, oncology clinics, psychiatry clinics, cardiac rehab places, and many other similar specialty type clinics.

Figure 4-1. Quality Improvement Using Plan-Do-Study-Act Cycle

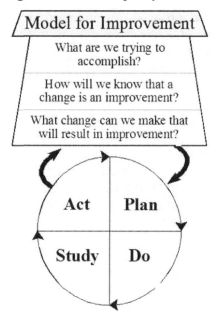

Figure 4-2. Quality Improvement Using Root Cause Analysis

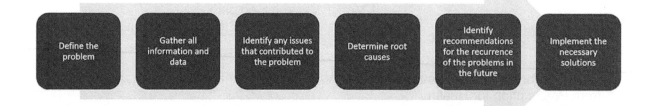

Table 4-20. Techniques for Root Cause Analysis:

Technique	How?
Five why's	Ask why five times to get to a root cause of an outcome
So what?	Ask about consequence to determine cause and effect
Fishbone Diagram	Head of fish: problem/effect; scales: each component of the process involved with branches including related possible causes and sub-causes of the problem/effect

CHAPTER 5
THE ROLE OF THE PRACTITIONER'S PERSONAL HEALTH AND COMMUNITY ADVOCACY

AMA Code of Medical Ethics: Physicians have a responsibility to maintain their health and wellness for the safety and effectiveness of the care they provide.

Table 5-1. Healthcare Provider Lifestyles

Unhealthy Behaviors	Healthy Healthcare Professionals
53% Moderate-Severe Stress	Doctors live longer than same race professionals in other occupations
53% Overweight or obese	Doctors (and medical students) exercise more than the public Nurses less likely to be obese
35% Insufficient exercise	
34 %Less than 6 hours of sleep	
27% No daily breakfast	Nurses more likely to meet dietary guidelines
13% Sedative use	
7% Depression	
4% Tobacco use	Health professionals have lower smoking rates than public
Higher alcohol use in nurses/healthcare professionals compared to general public	

Table 5-2. Impact of Practitioner Health on Patient Care

Own Health Practice	Effect
Doctors in overall good health	Healthy patients
Dietary habits	More counseling on low fat/low cholesterol, increasing fruits/vegetables
Exercising providers	High correlation with counseling frequency (OR 1.4-5.7)
Doctors who are actively improving own poor health	Counseled more than doctors NOT trying to improve self
Training doctors (tools, counseling resources)	Improves weight management care
Doctors with normal BMI	More physical activity counseling confidence
Non-smoking doctors	Discussed smoking risk more
Doctors with BMI less than patients'	Diagnose obesity more and counsel on weight loss
Screenings / vaccines /public health (seatbelts)	More likely to counsel on benefits; patients also more likely to comply by 14%.
Alcohol	Female physicians more likely to counsel on risks of alcohol use compared to male physicians

Table 5-3. Medical Staff Burnout

Definition	Long-term stress reaction marked by emotional exhaustion, depersonalization, and feelings of low personal satisfaction at work. Compassion fatigue - emotional, spiritual, or physical exhaustion from repeated or prolonged exposure to the suffering of others
Incidence	- 35-45% in nurses/physicians - 45-60% in medical students
Effect	Individuals may leave practice, reducing access to care in addition to potential patient safety and quality issues. These people can suffer from impaired attention, memory, and executive function.
Causes	Time pressure, documentation, loss of control, chaotic environment, home life.
How to Improve	Interventions must be BOTH individually focused and organizationally focused. These strategies include: flexible schedules, electronic record keeping and templates, more time to spend with patients, using team members such as nurses and medical assistants more effectively, surveys, system-wide quality improvement projects, and home life balance.

Therapeutic Alliance for all Healthcare Providers

Defined as "a measure of the (clinician's) and (patient's) mutual engagement in the work of (treatment)-thus representing an important component for achieving treatment success, regardless of the specific treatment modality employed."

Key Aspects:

- o Skillset and fortitude to initiate lifestyle changes in practice
- o Ability to "walk with" an individual and engage their support system
- o Ability to use educational and health coaching techniques
- o Maintain compassion (RAIN mneumonic): Recognize, Allow, Investigate, Nurture

Table 5-4. Practitioner Wellness

Personal	Integrate personal readiness assessment and SMART goals
Workplace	Examples include: 1) Wellness programs 2) On-site gym 3) Gym/health club discounts
Culture of Health	Examples include: 1) Healthy meals in and outside office, office events 2) Standing workstation or treadmill desk 3) Tracking technology (pedometer, apps) 4) Health challenges/competitions 5) Support of community events such as "Walk with a Doc"
Leadership	One of LM core competencies Interconnectivity with community Modeling personal health Professional Identity Formation-develop, embrace, and internalize the characteristics, values, and norms of their profession "Knowing, Doing, Being"
Benefits	Saving on healthcare costs, improving health, decreasing injuries, increasing productivity, and decreasing absenteeism.

Table 5-5. Practitioners as Advocates for Community-Level Change

Step 1	Understand your role/expertise
Step 2	Identify community needs/problems and determine priorities
Step 3	Set a goal and provide credibility/information/solutions
Step 4	Develop a plan/strategy, keeping in mind legal issues, your audience, timeline
Step 5	Plan/host events, provide educational materials
Step 6	If comfortable, use your network, speak at community events, do media talks
Step 7	Evaluate outcomes and re-strategize

Lifestyle Medicine Programs:

- Robert Wood Johnson: "Creating a Culture of Health"
- Dean Ornish: plant-based cardiac rehab covered by Medicare
- Blue Zones Project: community led collaboration
- Plan4Health Initiative: building local spaces for improving health
- Project for Public Spaces: NY and Kaiser Permanante
- Urban Land Institute: community design project for health
- Mainstreet America: Four Points (design, promotion, organization, economic vitality)
- Creative Placemaking: using art to transform communities
- National Complete Streets Coalition: safe street design

CHAPTER 6
NUTRITION SCIENCE

Table 6-1. U.S. Diet Changes Over the Last 100 Years

What Changed	Then	Now
Sugar in diet	< 10 lbs/yr	> 150 lbs/yr
Oil in diet	4 lbs/yr	70 lbs/yr
Cheese in diet	< 10 lbs/yr	38 lbs/yr

Table 6-2. Current U.S. Diet Trend

% of U.S. Diet	Content of Typical U.S. Diet
63%	Processed foods
25%	Animal foods
6%	Processed plant foods
6%	Unprocessed plant foods

Snacking instead of family meals, high-fructose corn syrup, meat and dairy (more available and cheaper because of industrial farming), larger portions and higher calorie counts, fast foods, increased intake of grains, oil, fats, and supplements.

Figure 6-1. Dietary Guidelines for Americans (2020-2025)

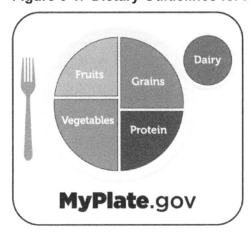

Table 6-3. Dietary Guidelines for Americans (DGA)

Issued by	U.S. Department of Agriculture & Department of Health and Human Services	Updated every five years (most recent 2020-2025)
Recommendations made by	Dietary Guidelines Advisory Committee (DGAC)	Nutrition and medical researchers
Influenced by	Public comments and public nominations to the committee	May allow for industry and special interests to have a role in crafting guidelines
Limitation example 1	Dairy recommendation not clear from infographic	Meant to represent calcium rich foods (could be soy based or fermented dairy)*
Limitation example 2	Cholesterol recommendation	Advise as little as possible (but no numerical limit given due to inadequate evidence that elevated dietary cholesterol causes CVD)*

See Table 6-6 for more discussion of dairy/saturated fat and cholesterol

Table 6-4. Global Dietary Guidelines Comparison

Meta-epidemiologic study of 78 clinical practice guidelines from 2010-2021 (Cara et al. Adv Nutrition 2023)	
Food most frequently encouraged (in order)	**Food most frequently discouraged (in order)**
Vegetables	Red meat
Fruits	Processed meat
Whole grains	Refined grains/desserts
Legumes/pulses	Fatty meat
Nuts/seeds	
Low fat dairy	
Seafood	

Table 6-5. Macronutrient Basics

The Good	Macronutrient	The Bad
Complex, low glycemic index	Carbohydrates (4 kcal/g)	Simple, high glycemic index
PUFAs and MUFAs	Fats (9 kcal/g)	Saturated, Trans
Vegetable based	Proteins (4 kcal/g)	Animal based

(Alcohol 7 kcal/g)

Figure 6-2. Carbohydrates

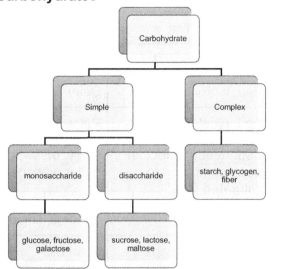

RDA 130g/day, main energy source for brain; prefer whole food/unrefined/natural sugars

- Carbohydrate
  - Simple
    - monosaccharide
      - glucose, fructose, galactose
    - disaccharide
      - sucrose, lactose, maltose
  - Complex
    - starch, glycogen, fiber

Figure 6-3. Fat

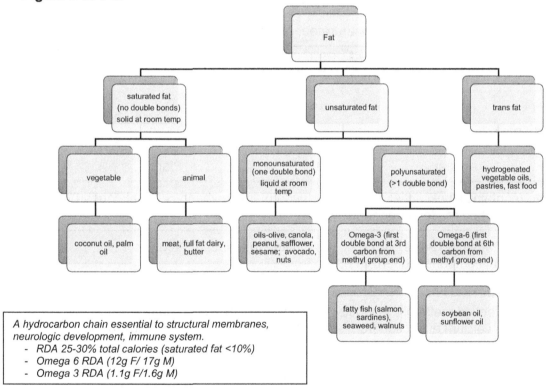

- Fat
  - saturated fat (no double bonds) solid at room temp
    - vegetable
      - coconut oil, palm oil
    - animal
      - meat, full fat dairy, butter
  - unsaturated fat
    - monounsaturated (one double bond) liquid at room temp
      - oils-olive, canola, peanut, safflower, sesame; avocado, nuts
    - polyunsaturated (>1 double bond)
      - Omega-3 (first double bond at 3rd carbon from methyl group end)
        - fatty fish (salmon, sardines), seaweed, walnuts
      - Omega-6 (first double bond at 6th carbon from methyl group end)
        - soybean oil, sunflower oil
  - trans fat
    - hydrogenated vegetable oils, pastries, fast food

A hydrocarbon chain essential to structural membranes, neurologic development, immune system.
- RDA 25-30% total calories (saturated fat <10%)
- Omega 6 RDA (12g F/ 17g M)
- Omega 3 RDA (1.1g F/1.6g M)

Table 6-6. Types of Fatty Acids

Name of Fatty Acid	Type of Fat	Most Common Food Sources
Lauric Acid	Saturated, high cholesterol	Coconuts
Myristic Acid	Saturated, high cholesterol	Dairy, tropical oils
Palmitic Acid	Saturated, most common	Palm oil, dairy, meat, cocoa
Stearic Acid	Saturated, neutral effect on cholesterol compared to other saturated fats	Dairy, meat-poultry, cocoa butter, chocolate
Oleic Acid	Monounsaturated	Olive oil, liquid oils
Linolenic acid	Polyunsaturated, omega 6	Plant oils
Arachidonic acid (AA)*	Polyunsaturated, omega 6	Meat
Alpha-linolenic acid (ALA)*	Polyunsaturated, omega 3	Plant oils, walnuts, flax
DHA/EPA	Polyunsaturated, omega 3	Cold water fish, seaweed

*There are pro- and anti-inflammatory properties in both omega 3 and 6 fats, but generally AA leads to pro-inflammatory cascade and ALA leads to anti-inflammatory cascade.

Table 6-7. Protein

Animal	Plant
Complete (contains all essential amino acids that cannot be made endogenously)	Incomplete (soybean is the exception)
All nine essential amino acids (major structural component of enzymes and hormones)	Limited in lysine, methionine
Possible diet-derived metabolic acidosis that can cause calcium extraction from bones to neutralize	**If a variety of whole plants consumed, protein content is adequate to meet needs**
Chicken, fish, beef, egg, yogurt, dairy	Soybean, oats, walnuts, corn, chickpea, baked potato, peas

RDA 0.8g/kg (~46g F/56g M); Special populations may have increased requirement: elderly, children, pregnancy, athletes

Figure 6-4. Understanding the Nutrition Label and Calculations

Unregulated packaging claims-natural, low sugar
Regulated packaging claims-good source (10-19% DV), excellent source (>20% DV), gluten-free, certified organic
%DV (daily value) <5% considered low, >20% considered high

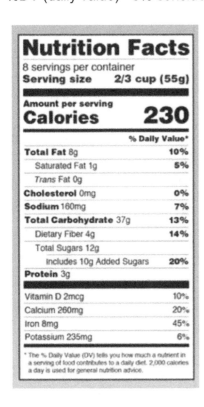

Fat = 8 g, so 8 x 9 kcals = 72 kcals

72/230 = 31% fat

Sugar = 12 g, so 12 x 4 kcals = 48 kcals

48/230 = 21% sugar

Fiber = 4 g, but 0 kcals

(25-30 g recommended)

4/25 = 16%   4/30 = 13%

Table 6-8. Overconsumed Nutrients

	Daily Guidelines*	Types	US Avg Intake*	Food Sources
Sugar	WHO/DGA: Limit <10% (12.5 tsp or 50g), Goal <5% AHA: Men 9 tsp (36g), Women 6 tsp (24g)	Cane sugar, HFCS (high fructose corn syrup), sucrose, fructose, dextrose, lactose, maltose, brown sugar, turbinado sugar, honey, agave, molasses, coconut sugar	~14% (18 tsp or 72g)	Fruit juice, sports drinks, baked goods/desserts, canned sauces and dressings, snack bars, cereal, jams and jellies
Cholesterol	NIH: <300mg DGA: as little as possible Key may be saturated fat in cholesterol containing foods	Triglycerides, Low density lipoprotein (LDL), very low density lipoprotein (VLDL), high density lipoprotein (HDL)	<300mg	Animal foods only-organ meats, egg yolk, animal meat (red meat>white meat>seafood), dairy (low fat better). (Egg yolk and shrimp are high in cholesterol but low in saturated fat)
Saturated Fat	DGA: <10% (22g) AHA: <5% (11g)	Saturated fat (no double bonds, typically solid at room temperature) vs monounsaturated fatty acid (MUFA) and polyunsaturated fatty acid (PUFA)	12% (26g)	Fatty cuts of meat, salami/sausage, processed meat, butter, cheese, coconut/palm oil. Cheese is top source due to volume consumed, even though fatty meat has more saturated fat per serving.
Sodium	DGA: <2300mg (1 tsp) <1500mg in some chronic conditions (HTN)	Restaurants/processed 70% Inherent to food 15% Added to food at home 5% Added at the table 5% Jeff Novick tip: look for sodium < calories per serving	3400mg	Commercially prepared foods especially burgers, tacos, sandwiches, pasta, rice, pizza, meats, soups
Trans Fat	0% FDA mandated removal in 2018	Unsaturated fat-natural and artifical forms	2%	Partially hydrogenated plant oils in many processed foods are main concern (baked goods, microwave popcorn, fast/fried food). Trace amounts found in meat and dairy products.

*% based on 2000 kcal daily diet
(Sources: WHO-World Health Organization, DGA-Dietary Guidelines for Americans, AHA-American Heart Association
Xu, A. (2018) Dietary Cholesterol Intake and Sources Among US Adults: Results from National health and Nutrition Examination Surveys (NHANES), 2001-2014. *Nutrients*, *10(6)*, 771.
https://www.ncbi.nlm.nih.gov/pmc/articles/PMC6024549/
Shan Z. (2019) Trends in dietary carbohydrate, protein, and fat intake and diet quality among US adults, 1999-2016. *JAMA*, *322*, 1178-1187.)

Table 6-9. Under consumed Nutrients (by ≥ 5% of Population or in Specific Groups)

	Recommended Dietary Allowance	Top Food Sources per serving (in order from highest to lowest)	US Avg Intake	Absorption	Notes
Calcium	19-50yr: 1000mg 51-70yr: 1000mg (M), 1200mg (F) 71+: 1200mg	Yogurt, foritfied orage juice, cheese, sardines, milk, fortified soymilk, tofu, salmon, soybeans, fortified cereal, spinach, turnip greens, kale, chia seeds, bok choi, beans	Men: 1083mg Women: 842mg	30% if from dairy, fortified foods, low-oxalate vegetables 5% if from high-oxalate vegetables Also affected by vitamin D	Certain compounds (oxalic acid, phytic acid) can decrease calcium absorption due to formation of indigestable salts. Ex: Spinach, collard greens, beet greens, swiss chard, sweet potatoes, rhubarb and beans
Fiber	Men: 30-38g (ideal 40g) Wome: 20-25g (ideal 45g) AHA: 25-30g	Wheat/bran cereal, artichoke, beans, split peas, lentils, pumpkin, brussel sprouts, sweet potato, berries, pear, popcorn, avocado, apple with skin, coconut, dried fig, flaxseed, oatmeal, bulgur, whole wheat pasta, brown rice, whole grain bread, almonds, peanuts	15g	Insoluble fiber (bran, vegetables, whole grains) increase stool bulk Soluble (viscous) fiber (oats, beans, psyllium) forms a gel, slows digestion, lowers cholesterol	*Fiber is found exclusively in plants Essential to a healthy gut microbiome. Also called prebiotic, fiber is a food source for intestinal bacteria, who then produce short chain fatty acids (postbiotics) which are anti-inflammatory and maintain the intestinal barrier
Magnesium	Men: 400-420mg Women: 310-320mg	Pumpkin seeds, chia seeds, brazil nuts, almonds, spinach, cashews, peanuts, cereal, soymilk, edamame, amaranth, potato, brown rice, yogurt, oatmeal, other nuts, tofu, black eyed peas, lima beans	150-200mg	30-40% consumed is absorbed	Generally, magnesium is found with fiber

Table 6-9 (cont.). Under consumed Nutrients (by ≥ 5% of Population or in Specific Groups)

Potassium	Men: 3400mg Women: 2600mg	Beet greens, beans, baked potato, acorn squash, spinach, apricots, lentils, prunes, kidney beans, soybeans, banana, milk, chicken, yogurt, salmon, cashews, tuna, coffee	Men: 2400mg Women: 1800mg	85-90% consumed is absorbed	Milk, coffee, tea and potatoes are current top sources
Vitamin A	Men: 900mcg RAE (retinol activity equivalents) Women: 700mcg RAE	Beef liver, sweet potato, spinach, carrot, canteloupe, butternut squash, dairy and plant fortifed milk, fortified cereal	Men: 680mcg RAE Women: 610mcg RAE	75-100% preformed (animal sources) 10-30% carotenoids (plant sources)	Fat soluble retinoid, critical for vision and immune health
Vitamin C	Men: 90mg Women: 75mg	Bell peppers, orange, grapefruit, kiwi, broccoli, strawberries, brussels, cabbage, tomato	RDAs generally met	70-90% (but falls with higher doses)	Water soluble
***Vitamin D**	19-70yr: 600 IU/15mcg 80yr+: 800 IU/20mcg 1 mcg = 40 IU	Trout, salmon, tuna (and other fish), mushrooms, soymilk, sardines, milk/yogurt, fortified orange juice, fortified cereal, egg, cheese	200 IU/5mcg	2 steps to active form: Liver-hydroxylation to 25(OH)D (used in serum measurement) Kidney-hydroxylation to 1,25(OH)D (physiologically active)	Produced endogenously by UV light exposure. Most of our Vit D needs are met through 20-30 min sun exposure 2x/wk Promotes calcium absorption in gut. Fat soluble.
Vitamin E	15mg	Wheat germ, sunflower seeds, almonds, plant oils, hazelnuts, peanuts, spinach, broccoli, kiwi, mango, tomato	Estimates are lower than RDA but don't consider cooking oils	Caution with low fat diets	Group of fat soluble antioxidants, alpha-tocopherol most important in humans
Choline	Men: 550mg Women: 425mg	Beef, egg, soybean, chicken, fish, potato, beans quinoa, yogurt, brussels, broccoli, mushrooms	M: 400mg W: 275mg	Absorption rates from different sources unknown	Body's main source of methyl groups for metabolism, can be produced by liver

(Sources: WHO-World Health Organization, DGA-Dietary Guidelines for Americans, AHA-American Heart Association)
*Deficiency is <12ng/ml
+Leafy greens contains vitamin K (coumadin interaction possible, consistency is key)

Evidence base and key studies:

See Key Studies (Chapter 13) and Tables 2-3 and 2-4 in Introduction to Lifestyle Medicine (Chapter 2)

Table 6-10. Food Processing

Type of Processing	Method and Impact
Removal of desired nutrients	Refinement of grains (removal of bran and germ removes iron, fiber, B vitamins) ex: white flour, white rice Dehydration Trimming, peeling, cutting
Addition of undesired ingredients	Artificial coloring (sweets) Sodium nitrite (deli meat) Artificial sweeteners (aspartame, sucralose, saccharin) Added sugar, salt or oils Saturated or trans fat
Food preparation	Canning (reduces water soluble vitamins like C and B) Drying (reduces vitamin C) Freezing (reheating may cause vitamin B/C loss) Boiling, simmering, poaching (nutrient loss) Frying (degrades PUFAs, promotes AGE formation *see Fig 6-5) Grilling/broiling (formation of AGEs, carcinogens like PAH) Roasting/baking (some nutrient loss)
Ultra-Processed Foods (UPFs)	Made through industrial methods and techniques, addition of ingredients to make foods hyperpalatable

*Not always negative (pasteurization, freezing, nutrient and vitamin fortification)

Inflammation-process by which the immune system recognizes and removes harmful and foreign stimuli and begins the healing process

Oxidation-chemical reaction in which an electron is lost from one substance to another; the generation of reactive oxygen species (ROS) and other free radicals in a normal metabolic process that ideally is compensated for by an endogenous antioxidant system

Glycosylation-biochemical process whereby a carbohydrate chain attaches to a protein/lipid/other organic molecule creating a glyconjugate; implicated in inflammatory response, viral immune escape, metastasis, apoptosis

Epigenetics-heritable changes of gene expression that are independent of DNA sequence and are reversible(methylation, histone modification, gene silencing)

Figure 6-5. Advanced Glycation End Products Formation

AGEs are formed by spontaneous chemical reaction between an amino acid (protein) and a monosaccharide (glucose). Major cause of oxidative stress and inflammation.

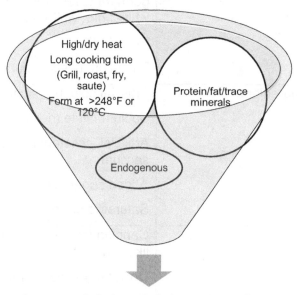

AGEs build up over time especially in protein in the lens of eye and collagen in skin; Directly related to T1DM, T2DM, atherosclerosis, kidney disease, poor wound healing

Table 6-11. Advanced Glycation End (AGE) Products in Food (AGE/serving)

Whole foods	10 (carrot)	799 (dried fig)
Processed food	17 (Snickers)	1522 (French fries)
Animal products	515 (smoked salmon)	11,905 (bacon-fried)
Dairy products	1 (fat free milk)	325 (heavy cream)
Nuts/seeds	753 (raw sunflower seeds)	3363 (roasted pine nuts)

(Source: Uribarri et al. Advanced Glycation End Products in Foods and a Practical Guide to their Reduction in the Diet, Jnl Aca Nutr and Diet, 2010;110(6). https://doi.org/10.1016/j.jada.2010.03.018.)

Table 6-12. Nutrition and Inflammation

Increases inflammatory mediators	Decreases oxidative stress (via antioxidants)	
Processed grain/sugar	Cruciferous vegetables	Sulphuraphane and indole-3 carbinols
Processed meat-group 1 carcinogen*	Dark berries/fruit	Polyphenols
Red meat-probable carcinogen (controversial)	Allium vegetables (garlic, onion, leek)	Organosulfurs
Trans fat, oxidized fat, solid/saturated fat	Orange/yellow fruits/vegetables	Carotenoids
Alcohol-group 1 carcinogen*	Dark leafy greens	High in K, Ca, Mg

Other Group 1 carcinogens: aflatoxinl, benzene, coal-tar, formaldehyde, hepatitis B/C, tobacco, radiation.

Microbiome-collective genomes of all microorganisms inhabiting an environment
Gut microbiome produces *short-chain fatty acids*, most importantly *butyrate*, also called postbiotics. Most common microbiota are: Bacteroidetes, Firmicutes, Actinobacteria, Proteobacteria, and Verrucomicrobia.
Microbiome support-Diversity of plants in diet, fermented foods, fiber-rich foods, complex carbohydrates and resistant starches, breastfeeding, plant-based diet with whole grains.
Microbiome disruptors-Fatty infiltration of pancreas, muscle, liver; antibiotics; low-fiber diet.
A healthy gut microbiome is associated with lower risk of CVD, DM2, cancer (many types but especially colon) and better mental health.

Table 6-13. Nutrition Advice

Encourage nutrient dense foods with maximum under consumed nutrients and minimum overconsumed nutrients	Vegetables, herbs/spices, fruits, legumes, whole grains, nuts/seeds Plants have antioxidant phytonutrients
Limit calorie dense/nutrient-poor foods	Sugar sweetened drinks, desserts, sandwiches with processed meat, tropical plant oils, butter/lard, fried food, red meat, refined grains, alcohol
Consider "food package" over specific macro/micronutrients	Ex: Milk and cheese are high in calcium but also saturated fat→is there a better way to get calcium?
Choose whole foods (no or minimal processing)	Ex: Apple→peeled without skin→applesauce→apple juice→apple flavoring in candy/baked dessert
"Eat food, mostly plants, not too much" *(Michael Pollen)*	Focus on whole foods, predominately plants, in appropriate portions
Eat the rainbow	A variety of colors indicates a variety of phytonutrients (flavonoids, vitamins) and should be adequate to meet most RDAs (may need B12 and vitamin D supplements)

Culinary Medicine
Combines nutrition science and culinary science; skill-based teaching; curriculum available for medical school/residency use and nutrition course instructors to improve practitioner knowledge and self-efficacy so they can counsel patients effectively.

Table 6-14. Components of Nutrition Prescription

Positive prescription	Eat more of "x"	Vegetable, legumes
Negative prescription	Eat less of "x"	Dessert, processed meat
Swap prescription	Swap "x" for "y"	Cook with olive oil instead of butter
Specific	Exact food	Spinach (vs. vegetable)
Measurable	Portion	1 cup
Achievable	Who does the cooking, where will you eat?	Buy prewashed bag and serve with dinner nightly
Realistic	Small steps	One or two small changes at a time (vs complete overhaul)
Time	Frequency; for how long?	Nightly for two weeks
Role of Registered Dietitian	Assess/monitor Use PES format (Problem, Etiology, Signs/symptoms) Determine macro/ micronutrient needs Individualized plans Coaching	Refer when: 2+ chronic conditions, liquid meals necessary, on weight-modulating medications, not responding to initial nutritional intervention

All prescriptions should have patient's name, date, and signature of provider.

Table 6-15. Nutrition Assessment (ABCD)

Anthropometric data	Weight, height, BMI, waist circumference (less common: body composition)
Biochemical data	Labs (see Chapter 4)
Clinical assessment	History and physical, including activity level and nutrition history
Dietary assessment (this may be assigned to a registered dietitian (RD)	Daily intake, 24hr recall, 3-day food diary, Mini Nutritional Assessment (MNA) for the elderly
	Tracking tools from Nutrition Quest, CDC, commercial apps
	Ask about schedule, portions, method of food prep, snacks, supplements, drinks
	Consider psychosocial history-knowledge, cultural preferences/restrictions, finances, emotions/motivation

*Physician may have supervising role (create framework, lead team); RD may individualize and track progress.

Table 6-16. Advantages of a Whole Food, Plant-Based Diet

- Reduction in BMI (BROAD study-compared to Western diet) (New DIETs trial suggests vegan superior); decreased calorie intake and reduced hunger craving
- Reduced risk T2DM, improved glucose homeostasis, improved insulin sensitivity, reverses diabetic retinopathy, protects pancreatic beta cells from injury
- Lower risk all cause and cardiovascular related mortality, reduced incidence of stroke/CAD, reduction in cardiovascular risk factors like hypertension, hyperlipidemia (CARDIVEG study)
- Decreases colorectal cancer risk
- Reduced risk Alzheimer's disease (MAP study)
- Decreases inflammatory mediators like CRP
- Optimizes microbiome and short-chain fatty acid production
- Changes epigenetics
- Decreases pain of peripheral neuropathy (80% of sufferers improved within two weeks)
- Tastes can be changed within two weeks to crave less refined foods and lower glycemic load, thereby helping with food addiction
- Phytochemicals help normalize dopamine reward system

Foundational Elements of Diet Prescriptions for Chronic Diseases:

- Whole foods, plant-predominant
- Vegetables/fruits (5 servings daily)
- Legumes
- Whole grains and pulses
- Nuts and seeds
- High in fiber and antioxidants
- Low in saturated fat, added sugar, added salt

Table 6-17. Plant Predominant Dietary Plans Used in Research

Mediterranean Diet	- Monounsaturated > saturated fats - High in legumes, fruits, vegetables, grains/cereals - Moderate in red wine and dairy - Fish > red meat intake	- Improved BP, TGL, and cholesterol - May decrease CV events, incidence of T2DM and breast ca
Dietary Approaches to Stop Hypertension (DASH)	- Low in sodium, saturated/trans fats, and added sugars - Focus on fruits, vegetables, whole grains, low fat dairy, fish, poultry, beans, nuts, vegetable oils - Focus on K, Ca, Mg, fiber, and protein	- Improved BP, weight management - Lower stroke, CAD, and heart failure incidence
Med.-DASH Intervention for Neurodegenerative Delay (MIND)	Combination of Mediterranean and DASH	May be protective against development of Alzheimer's
Portfolio Diet	High in plant sterols, soy protein, viscous fibers, almonds & Low in saturated fat	Lowered LDL = to statin (~30%)

CARDIOVASCULAR DISEASE

Table 6-18. Nutrition Recommendations

Reduce Intake of	Increase Intake of
Hypertension	
Sodium *< 2300mg/day; AHA goal < 1500mg/day (see DASH diet Table 2-4)* *(Common sources: pizza, snacks, sandwiches, canned foods)*	Potassium *(Common sources: potatoes, cantaloupe, bananas, squash, broccoli, spinach, legumes)*
Caffeine	Calcium *(Common sources: leafy greens, white beans, fortified nut milks)*

Alcohol
    < 1 drink/day in women
    < 2 drinks/day in men
	Magnesium
	(Common sources: almonds, cashews, beans, amaranth, quinoa, avocado)

	Garlic
Hyperlipidemia	
Trans/saturated Fats *(Common sources: cheese, butter, high fat dairy, processed and animal protein; butter increases LDL the most of these)*	Unsaturated fats
Processed foods	Complex carbohydrates
Animal products (especially total meat intake)	Plant sterols/viscous fiber *(Common sources: oats, soy, peas, legumes, eggplant, okra, almonds, wheat germ)*

Water-only fasting: Water only fasting can lower BP but perform *only under medical supervision*

Table 6-19. Evidence for Nutrition Recommendations

Study	Intervention	Outcome
Effects of stress management training and dietary changes in treating ischemic heart disease *(Ornish 1983)*	See Key Study #1	- 91% reduction in anginal episodes - 44% increase in exercise tolerance
Angina pectoris and atherosclerotic risk factors in the multisite cardiac lifestyle intervention program *(Frattoroli 2008)*	10% fat diet, exercise, and stress management effect on angina	- At 12 weeks, 74% were symptom-free - Similar results to CABG and PCI procedures
Updating a 12-year experience with arrest and reversal therapy for coronary heart disease (an overdue requiem for palliative cardiology). T(1999) A way to reverse CAD? *(Esselstyn 2014)*	Whole-food, plant-based diet, oil-free, no meat, only skim milk and non-fat yogurt	- No CVD extension, coronary events, or cardiac interventions over 12 years if adherent - Case series on 198 patients with similar diet (w/o dairy) had 0.6% cardiac events vs. 62% in 21 non-adherent pts

See also: Jenkins "Portfolio Diet" study (#9) and Ornish Lifestyle Heart Trial (#1) in Key Studies.

Table 6-20. Epidemiology and Effect of Plant-Based Diets

Mechanisms of Plant-Based Atherosclerosis Reversal	- Improved vascular function, plaque dissolution; angina reduction - Antioxidants reduce inflammation and reactive nitrogen species - Average LDL in vegans (69) vs. omnivores (123) *(De Biase et al. Vegetarian diet and cholesterol and triglyceride levels 2007)* - HDL may dec on plant-based diet, but ratio LDL/HDL improves - Trans fats raise CVD risk regardless of origin
Plant-Based Cultures*	- Tarahumara, Papua New Guinea, rural China, rural Africa - Diets rich in beans, corn, sweet potatoes, green plantains, rice/vegetables and have very low rates of CVD
Diet, Lifestyle and Etiology of CAD *(Campbell 1998)*	- Higher fiber, 1/10th meat intake of U.S - Lower cholesterol, 16.7-fold less CAD mortality in men
2013 Baylor University Conference	- Cholesterol is the main risk factor for heart disease - TC goal levels: 90-140 to eliminate risk of atherogenic plaques - Optimal LDL: 50-70, Atherosclerosis does not advance if LDL < 70 - 75% of heart attacks fell into "normal" LDL range

*(Sources: *Shaper et al. Serum-cholesterol, diet, and coronary heart-disease in Africans and Asians in Uganda. Int J Epidemiol, 2012;41(5):1221-1225. ; Connor et al. The plasma lipids, lipoproteins, and diet of the Tarahumara Indians of Mexico. Am J Clin Nutr, 1978;31(7):1131-1142. ; Sinnett et al. Epidemiological studies in a total highland population, Tukisenta, New Guinea. J Chronic Dis, 1973; 26(5):262-290.; Facts and principles learned at the 39th Annual Williamsburg Conference on Heart Disease. https://www.ncbi.nlm.nih.gov/pmc/articles/PMC3603726/pdf/bumc0026-0124.pdf)*

TYPE 2 DIABETES MELLITUS (T2DM)

Table 6-21. Nutrition Recommendations

Reduce Intake of:	Increase Intake of:
Saturated and trans fats *(Common sources: cheese, high fat dairy, animal protein)*	Fiber *(Common sources: legumes, vegetables, fruits, whole grains)*
Simple and processed sugars	
Processed grains *(Common sources: baked goods, snacks)*	
High glycemic foods *(Common sources: white bread, rice, potatoes, ice cream, fruit yogurt)*	Low glycemic foods *(Common sources: bran cereal, vegetables, soybeans, nuts)*

Table 6-22. Evidence for Nutrition Recommendations

Study	Intervention	Outcome
Adventist Health Study-2 Usefulness of vegetarian and vegan diets for treating T2DM *(Barnard 2010)*	Vegetarian diets: - Associated with decreased diabetes prevalence - Improved BMI	Prevalence of T2DM: - Non-vegetarian - 1.0 - Semi-vegetarian - 0.72 - Pesco-vegetarian - 0.49 - Lacto-ovo-vegetarian - 0.39 - Vegan - 0.22
High-carbohydrate, high-fiber diets for insulin-treated men with diabetes mellitus *(Anderson 1979)*	- High-fiber, plant-based diet (65g/d) in 20 men w/ T2DM - Sufficient calories, so no weight loss	Insulin stopped or reduced in all within two weeks
Glycemic and cardiovascular parameters improved in T2DM with high nutrient dense (HND) diet *(Dunaief 2012)*	- Diet high in phytochemicals/ antioxidants from fruits, vegetables, legumes, and nuts/seeds - 13 patients	- HbA1c decreased 8.2% → 5.8% - Many stopped meds or decreased
A low-fat vegan diet and a conventional diabetes diet in the treatment of T2DM: a 74-wk of RCT *(Barnard 2009)*	(theoretical explanation)	Low-fat vegan diet found to be better diet quality than recommended ADA diet for diabetes

Table 6-23. Effects of Diet on T2DM

Type of Diet	Effects
Vegan vs ADA diet *A low fat vegan diet improves glycemic control and cardiovascular risk factors in a randomized clinical trial in individuals with type 2 diabetes. (Barnard 2006)*	- Healthy low-fat vegan diet may be better for weight loss, decrease in fasting glucose, and reduction of medications. - Plant based diet was 3x better in reducing HbA1c, and 2x better in improving LDL, weight loss, and decreasing medications. - Barnard's 2008 study showed greater reductions in HbA1c levels. These effects were sustained at a one-year follow-up.
Plant-based dietary patterns and incidence of T2DM in U.S. men and women: results from three prospective cohort studies. (Satija 2016)	- Processed plant-based diet led to 16% increased risk of T2DM compared to healthy plant-based diet
Vegetarian diet vs ADA *Vegetarian diet improves insulin resistance and oxidative stress markers more than conventional diet in. subjects with type 2 diabetes. (Kahleova 2011)*	- In those with T2DM, vegetarians lost more weight and reduced medication more than those on ADA diet. - 2018 Rotterdam Study (Chen et al) showed that the higher the score on the plant-based dietary index, the lower was insulin resistance and risk of T2DM.
Mediterranean diet	- Reduces risk of developing T2DM by 20-30% and improves both insulin sensitivity and HbA1c.
Meat and T2DM *(Nurses Health Study; Red meat consumption and risk type 2 diabetes, Pan et al 2011)*	- Eating processed meats five or more times/wk increased risk of T2DM. - Diabetes risk decreases by 16-35% if one meat meal is replaced with one meal with nuts, grains, or low-fat dairy.
Eggs and T2DM *(Nurses Health Study and Health Professionals Study-see Table 2-3 for more info))*	- Eating eggs > 5 days/wk increases risk of DM (may be due to inflammation from carnitine and choline). - Eating eggs > 7 days/wk doubles risk of heart disease in those already with T2DM.
Fiber and T2DM	- Regular dietary fiber intake is associated with lower all-cause mortality in people with T2DM. - The ADA recommends that fiber be incorporated through foods that are naturally high in fiber, as opposed to relying on supplements.

Note: Weight loss leads to decreased inflammation and increased insulin sensitivity.

Table 6-24. Studies of Diet and Therapy for T2DM

Study	Findings

Nurses' Health Study	- 91% of the risk of T2DM is due to five factors:
	  o BMI > 25 (strongest predictor)
	  o Poor diet (low in fiber, low in polyunsaturated fat, high in trans fat, high glycemic load)
	  o Inactivity
	  o Smoking
	  o More than one-half of an alcoholic drink/day
	- Among drinks:
	  o Coffee lowered risk
	  o Sugar-sweetened beverages and juice increased risk

Adventist Health Study	- Eating meat, especially processed meat, doubled risk of T2DM - 80% higher prevalence in meat-eating men - 40% higher prevalence in meat-eating women - 97% increased risk of T2DM in Adventist men who ate meat compared to other Adventists - 93% increased risk of T2DM in Adventist women who ate meat compared to other Adventists
EPIC-InterAct Study	- Every 5% of protein from animals was associated with 30% increase in T2DM - Intake of all forms of dairy products was not related to future diabetes risk, but fermented dairy product intake was associated with a reduced risk of diabetes - Highest fruit and vegetable intake had a 7% lower risk of diabetes, with a particular benefit linked to consumption of green leafy vegetables
Gastric Bypass and T2DM *(STAMPEDE study and Swedish Obese Subjects follow-up studies)*	- Remission rates at five years were 29% in STAMPEDE study and 30% at 15 years in Swedish Obese Subjects study - Both studies identified weight loss, a decrease in need for medication by 9-30%, and a decrease in all-cause mortality

Note: Patients should follow the diet that they feel they can adhere to best.

Table 6-25. Diabetes Management

Medical management	Current approach is aimed at delaying progression, but not cure
Lifestyle management	Lifestyle factors (weight, BP, low HDL, high triglycerides, inactivity) are the cause of and the cure for T2DM
ACCORD study	2008 intensive medical trial which had a primary goal to lower glucose actually increased mortality and did not significantly reduce major cardiovascular events
Insulin side effects	Weight gain, hypoglycemia, lipodystrophy, hypokalemia, CHF, breast cancer, prostate cancer, colorectal cancer, and adverse drug interactions

Table 6-26. Diabetes Prevention Program: An Intensive Lifestyle Program to Reduce Progression of Prediabetes in High-Risk Patients

Program description *(first screen high-risk patients with labs and questionnaires)*	- 12-month program (weekly x 6 months, then monthly). - Problem-solving and coping skills are taught. - Diet: "MyPlate" model of low-fat, low-calorie. - Exercise: Meet physical activity guidelines for Americans (150 minutes of moderate intensity/wk), usually with walking recommended.
Initial results	- Initial results: T2DM in at-risk adults was reduced by 58% with intensive lifestyle intervention, and by 31% with metformin, compared with placebo.
Follow-up results	- Incidence of diabetes remained lowest in the lifestyle group. - Prevention or delay of diabetes with lifestyle intervention or metformin can persist for at least 10 years.
Challenges	- Achieving goals hinges on intensity and duration of participation. - Identifying, engaging, and retaining those at risk.

Figure 6-6. Pathogenesis of T2DM

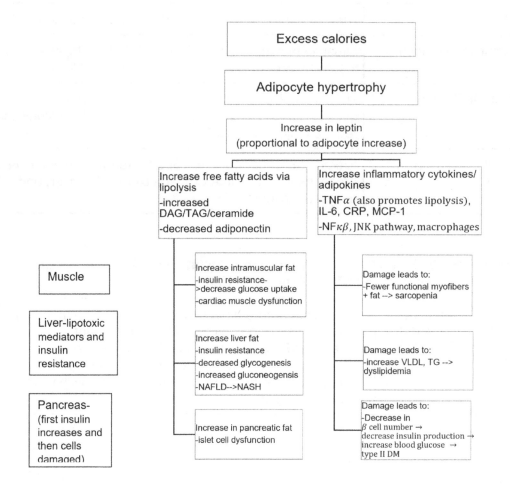

(Sources:
Nielsen, T.S. (2014) Dissecting adipose tissue lipolysis: molecular regulation and implications for metabolic disease. Jnl Mol Endocrin, 52(3), R199-222
Vachharajani, V. (2010) Adipose tissue: A motor for the inflammation associated with obesity. IUBMB Life, 61(4), 424-430.
De Ferranti S. (2008 Jun) The perfect storm: obesity, adipocyte dysfunction, and metabolic consequences. Clin Chem 54(6), 945-955.
Pico C. (2022) Leptin as a key regulator of the adipose organ. Reviews Endocr Met Dis, 23, 13-30.)

Table 6-27. Hormones Involved in T2DM

Hormone	Produced by	Action	Levels in Patients with Obesity
Leptin	Adipose tissue and small intestine	Decrease hunger (also proangiogenic)	High (resistant) Increased sugar craving
Ghrelin	Gastrointestinal tract	Increase hunger	Low
Insulin	Pancreatic β-cells	Decrease blood glucose -Muscle glycogenesis -Liver glycogenesis and lipogenesis -Fat lipogenesis	High (resistant)
Adiponectin	Primarily adipose tissue	Enhances insulin	Low
Glucagon	Pancreatic α-cells	Increase blood glucose -Liver glycogenolysis and gluconeogenesis	High

Table 6-28. Mediators of T2DM

Triacylglycerol	Fatty acids stored in and are damaging to muscle (low carb diet may not decrease intramyocellular lipids)
Gluconeogenesis	Fat deposits in liver make it unable to suppress more glucose being made by the liver
NF-K-beta pathway	- Free radicals and inflammation initiate this pathway, which is associated with aging, allergies, Alzheimer's, arthritis, asthma, atherosclerosis, autoimmune disease, cancer, colitis, diabetes, and GI disease - Phytonutrients and antioxidants, but not medications, downregulate this path
Role of macrophages	Part of the immune system that can kill beta cells and activate inflammatory paths
Heme iron *(in red meat)*	Pro-oxidant, proinflammatory, and increases insulin resistance
Dyslipidemia	VLDL and LDL can lead to beta cell death

CANCER

Table 6-29. Specific Site-Based Cancer Nutrition Recommendations

Cancer	Increase	Decrease
Breast Cancer	Soy, fruits, vegetables	Red meat, processed meat, extra calories, alcohol
Colon Cancer	Fiber, calcium, folate	Red meat, processed meat
Gastric Cancer	Fruits, vegetables	Processed meat
Prostate Cancer	Soy, lycopene, selenium	Red meat, processed meat

Table 6-30. Nutrition Recommendations

Reduce Intake of:	Increase Intake of:
Animal proteins and processed meat	Plant proteins/soybeans
Simple and processed sugars	Low glycemic foods *(Common sources: bran cereal, vegetables, soybeans, nuts)*
Processed grains- baked goods, snacks	Antioxidant-rich foods (whole foods preferable to supplements): - beta carotene *(carrot, sweet potato, spinach, kale)* - lycopene *(tomato, watermelon, grapefruit, guava)* - resveratrol *(red grapes, blueberries, peanuts, soy)* - selenium *(Brazil nuts, sunflower seeds, mushrooms, fish)* - vitamin C *(citrus, melon, berries)* - vitamin E *(almonds, peanuts, leafy greens)*
AGEs	Fiber goal: >30-35g/day

Table 6-31. Evidence for Nutrition Recommendations

Study	Intervention	Outcome
Clinical events in prostate cancer lifestyle trial *(Frattaroli 2008)*	Low-fat and plant-based diet, exercise, stress management, group support, 2 yrs	- Intervention: 2/43 needed treatment, 70% growth suppression of tumor cells - Control: 13/49 needed treatment in control, 9% suppression of tumor cells
Effects of low-fat, high-fiber diet and exercise program on breast cancer risk factors *(Bernard 2006)*	Low-fat and high-fiber diet, plus exercise - 12 women, 2 wks of intervention	- Reduced breast cancer cell growth - Increased apoptosis - Dec IGF-1 (inc in IGF-1 binding protein that removes it from blood)
Greater survival after breast ca in physically active women with high vegetable-fruit intake *(Pierce 2007)*	Five servings fruits/ vegetables daily and 180 min moderate exercise weekly	- 1490 women - 50% mortality risk reduction - Irrespective of obesity status if physically active

OTHER CHRONIC DISEASES

Table 6-32. Role of Nutrition in Other Chronic Diseases

Disease	Findings	Citation
Cataracts	Plant based diet lowers risk	Diet, vegetarianism, and cataract risk *(Appleby 2011)*
COPD	24% lower mortality with 100g increase in fruit daily	Diet and 20-year chronic obstructive pulmonary disease mortality in middle-aged men from three European countries *(Walda 2002)*
	Improvements in lung function testing with fruits and vegetables	Impact of dietary shift to higher-antioxidant foods in COPD: a randomized trial *(Keranis 2010)*
Kidney Disease	Animal protein, fat, and cholesterol all associated with decline in renal function and increased albuminuria	Associations of diet with albuminuria and kidney function decline *(Lin 2010)*
Immune Function	Higher response to vaccines in those with more plant intake	Effect of fruit and vegetable consumption on immune function in older people: a randomized controlled trial *(Gibson 2012)*
Crohn's Disease	Semi-vegetarian diet → 80% remission rate	Lifestyle-related disease in Crohn's disease: relapse prevention by a semi-vegetarian diet *(Chiba 2010)*
Multiple Sclerosis	Slower disease progression with restricted saturated fat intake	Is the treatment of multiple sclerosis headed in the wrong direction? *(Kadoch 2012)*

CHAPTER 7
OBESITY MEDICINE

"Obesity is defined as a chronic, progressive, relapsing, and treatable multi-factorial, neurobehavioral disease, wherein an increase in body fat promotes adipose tissue dysfunction and abnormal fat mass physical forces, resulting in adverse metabolic, biomechanical, and psychosocial health consequences." (Obesity Medicine Association)

Definitions:

Total energy expenditure: Resting energy expenditure (REE 60%) + Thermic effect of feeding (TEF 5-10%) + Non-resting energy expenditure (NREE 30-35%).

Adaptive thermogenesis (aka *plateau phenomenon*): Decrease in energy expenditure by increase in efficiency and decrease in REE stimulated by caloric restriction/weight loss.

Adiposopathy ("sick fat"): Pathogenic adipose tissue anatomic/functional derangements that result in adverse health conditions.

Metabolic syndrome: Not a disease, but a clustering of atherosclerotic cardiovascular risk factors; abdominal obesity, elevated triglycerides, low HDL, HTN, elevated fasting glucose.

Obesity paradox: Underweight patients may paradoxically have less favorable disease outcomes (confounding effects of poor nutrition, malabsorption, cancer, cigarette use).

Table 7-1. Clinical Manifestations of Obesity

Cardiovascular	CHF, cor pulmonale, HTN, varicose veins, thromboembolic events
Pulmonary	Dyspnea, asthma, obstructive sleep apnea, Pickwickian syndrome (hypoventilation)
Neurologic	Reduced grey matter, intracranial HTN (pseudotumor cerebri), stroke, nerve entrapment
Musculoskeletal	Immobility, osteoarthritis, back pain, myalgia, altered center of gravity, disequilibrium
Gastrointestinal	GERD, hernia, NAFLD
Integument	Venous stasis ulcers, cellulitis, carbuncles, skin infections, stretch marks
Genitourinary	Hormone dysregulation, infertility, incontinence, PCOS, pregnancy complications, pelvic organ prolapse
Psychosocial	Depression, diminished sex drive, decreased work productivity
Immune	Increased risk of cancer, acute respiratory virus infection

Diagnostic measures of obesity

See Table 4-4 and 4-5 for BMI, obesity staging and waist circumference

See Table 8-7 for percent body fat

Table 7-2. Treatment Options for Obesity

Comprehensive Lifestyle Intervention *(at least 6 months)*	Refer: - BMI ≥ 25 with CVD - BMI ≥ 30	Caloric restriction, physical activity, behavioral strategies Patients' expectations need to be addressed early
Weight Loss *(difficult to achieve with only physical exercise)*	Calorie reduction	M: Reduce by 750 cal/day to goal of 1500-1800 calories F: Reduce by 500 cal/day to goal of 1200-1500 calories
	Diet	No optimal diet (see Key Study #3), adherence is more important
	Increase NREE/physical activity	- 150-300 min moderate intensity; OR - 75-150 min vigorous intensity + resistance training at least 2x/wk
Pharmaceutical	Refer: - BMI ≥ 30 - BMI ≥ 27 with an obesity related comorbidity	Phentermine/topiramate, Orlistat, naltrexone/bupropion, liraglutide
		GLP-1 receptor agonist, weekly injectable, approved 2021
Bariatric Surgery	Refer: - BMI ≥ 40 - BMI ≥ 35 with an obesity related comorbidity	≈50% excess weight lost in first 6mon and can be maintained for >10yrs after surgery (O'Brien P.E. (2013) Long term outcomes after bariatric surgery. *Ann of Surg, 257(1)*, 87-94)

- Weight loss of 3-5% can improve glucose, HbA1c, triglycerides, and insulin resistance.
- Weight loss of >5% can improve HTN, lipid disorders, and reduce medications.
- Weight loss goal of 5-10% of body weight for overweight/obese patients (intensive lifestyle intervention on average reduces weight by 8kg or 17 pounds).

CHAPTER 8
PHYSICAL ACTIVITY AND EXERCISE SCIENCE

Table 8.1 Terms to Know

Term	Definition	Notes / Benefits
Physical Activity	Movement of the body through skeletal muscle contractions	
Physical Inactivity	Time not engaged in physical activity	Includes NEAT and sedentary time
NEAT	*Non-Exercise Activity Thermogenesis)*: Energy that is used for all non-exercise, non-eating, and non-sleeping activity	E.g. Fidgeting, housework, shopping, etc.
Sedentary Behavior	Low energy expenditure, usually <1.5 METs, for prolonged times	
Exercise	Organized, planned, and recurring purposeful activity	4 types: Strength, Flexibility, Balance, & Cardiorespiratory
Cardiorespiratory Fitness/Aerobic	Large muscles move rhythmically over time	Benefits: See Table 8-2
Strength/Resistance Training	Muscles contract against an external force (Tip: Avoid back-to-back same muscle group workouts.)	Improved bone density, inc lean body mass; reduce fatigue, injury, body fat, arthritis pain, hepatic steatosis; leads to better sleep, quality of life, cholesterol / lipids / glucose levels and insulin sensitivity
Flexibility	Ranging motion at a joint (Tip: Stretching best when done with warm muscles and daily.)	Improves range of motion and increases muscle length; helps heal muscles, hip flexor stretches increase gait and stride length in elderly
Balance (static and dynamic)	Ability to withstand destabilizing stimuli or postural sway	- dec in falls by: - 61% that led to fractures - 43% that led to severe injury - 30% decrease in injuries that need care*

(Source: *El-Khoury, F. (2013) The effect of fall prevention exercise programs on fall induced injuries in community dwelling older adults. BMJ https://doi.org/10.1136/bmj.f6234)

Cardiorespiratory fitness (CRF) or endurance training is superior to resistance exercise in all areas of physiologic improvement except lean body mass, muscle strength, and basal metabolic rate. Strength/Resistance Training is more efficient than CRF for bone and muscle strengthening.

Table 8-2. Benefits of Physical Activity

System	Benefit
General	- Lower risk of all causes of mortality (increased life expectancy at ALL levels of BMI and ANY amount of exercise), higher perceived quality of life, better sleep (onset, quality, duration), better cognition on day of exercise, reduced risk of obesity
Musculoskeletal	- Improved muscular and bone health - Less risk of falls (including vertebral falls) - Helps after limb amputations as well as mobility impairments, including scoliosis
Hematology/Oncology	- Reduced risk breast and colon cancer
Neurology/Psychology	- Helpful for depression, anxiety, dementia, intellectual disability, stroke, spinal cord injury, multiple sclerosis, muscular dystrophy, Parkinson's (stability best improved with tai chi over other alternatives), CP, traumatic brain injury
Cardiovascular	- Reduced hypertension and CVD - Improved lipids, especially reduction in triglycerides
Endocrinology	- Improved glucose metabolism, insulin sensitivity, and better weight management
Pediatric	- Improved cognitive and physical function, bone health, weight - Less depression
Geriatric	- Lower risk of falls and fall-related injuries - Better day-to-day functioning
Health Care Spending (*think "5"*)	- 1 day of exercise decreases costs by <u>5</u>% - $<u>5</u>00-$<u>5</u>,000 to get one inactive person to be active - Inactive person costs $1,<u>5</u>00 more than an active person *(Carlson SA.(2015) Inadequate Physical Activity and Health Care Expenditures in the United States. Prog Cardiovasc Dis; 57(4):315-323.)*

Table 8-3. The Dangers of Sitting

7% of all-cause mortality is associated with habitual prolonged sitting
Disease risk increases, **even if** sufficient exercise performed
Consistent among all ages, gender, chronic disease comorbidities
Walking breaks of 2 minutes every 20 minutes improves glucose and insulin levels
Watching TV associated with increased all-cause mortality even with seven hours of exercise/wk (same risk as no TV and no exercise)
Replacing 30 minutes of sitting per day with low-intensity physical activity lowers risk of early death by 17 percent
Reducing sitting time from 6 to 3 hours adds up to 2 years life expectancy
Switching to standing for just 2 hours/day is associated with 10% reduction in mortality.

*Standing: Per the ADA, breaking up prolonged sitting reduces the postprandial glucose and insulin in diabetics. **Standing desk** workers burn only a few more calories than those sitting; a treadmill desk is even better for energy expenditure.
(Source: Hidde P et al. (2012) Sitting Time and All-Cause Mortality Risk in 222,497 Australian Adults. Arch Intern Med; 172(6):494-500.)

Low cardiorespiratory fitness = #1 cause of preventable deaths from all-cause mortality.

Table 8-4. Exercise vs. Medication

		Meds	LM
Diabetes Prevention Program (LM vs. Metformin vs. Placebo)	Lifestyle (7% weight loss and 150 mins/wk exercise)	T2DM down by 31%	T2DM down by 58%
	Number needed to treat	14	7
Secondary prevention of CAD		Meds = Exercise	
Stroke rehabilitation		Meds < Exercise	
T2DM prevention (pre-DM)		Meds = Exercise	
Congestive Heart Failure		Meds > Exercise	
HTN		Meds > Exercise	

Table 8-5. Weekend Warrior (WW) – All exercise done in 1-2 days, usually vigorous

2004 study *	Men with no RFs	WW had a lower risk of dying than sedentary men
	Men with one or more risk factors	WWs did not decrease odds of dying; better to recommend space out exercise
2017 study **	Males and females	30% dec in all-cause mortality in all. The more moderate-vigorous exercise done, the lower the mortality rate. CRF of WWs only slightly worse than non-WWs. Injury higher in WWs.

* *Am J Epidemiol 2004 Oct 1;160(7):636-41. doi: 10.1093/aje/kwh274.*
** *JAMA Intern Med. 2017;177(3):335-342. doi:10.1001/jamainternmed.2016.8014*

Table 8-6 Exercise Terms

Term	Definition	Notes / Benefits
Fitness	Ability to do one's daily activities without fatigue	
Muscle Mass	Weight of the muscle	Muscle quality more important
Muscle Quality	Lower intramuscular fat content is higher quality muscle	
Metabolic Equivalent of a Task (MET):	The ratio of the rate at which a person uses energy (relative to their weight) during a task to a standard resting metabolic rate	See Table 8-9
Standard Resting Metabolic Rate	The amount of O_2 consumed during quiet rest/sitting; approximately 3.5 mL of O_2/kg/min (1 MET)	Also called Basal Metabolic Rate (BMR)
Repetitions (Reps)	The number of times a weight is lifted	
Sets	The number of cycles of repetitions	
Dynamic Stretching	Gradual increase in reach as movement is repeated	
Static Stretching	Slow reach, steady hold	-
Ballistic Stretching	Repetitive small bouncing movement (slow, low tension, use with caution)	-

Table 8-7. Special Population Recommendations

Population	Recommendations	Comments
Pregnant/ Postpartum	- Aerobic: 150 minutes of moderate intensity; If patient did vigorous pre-pregnancy exercise, can continue, but adjust in later pregnancy as needed - Resistance: Pelvic floor exercises	- Helps prevent weight gain, depression, GDM, preeclampsia, C-section, preterm labor, low birthweight infant - General concerns: avoid overheating, lying on - back in 3rd trimester (compresses vena cava), contact sports, activities with high risk of falling - Absolute contraindications: Restrictive lung disease, hemodynamically significant heart disease, incompetent cervix, multiple gestation (risk for preterm labor), 2nd or 3rd trimester bleeding, placenta previa after 26 weeks gestation, premature labor, ruptured membranes, or preeclampsia risk
Ischemic Heart Disease Prevention	- Even weekly low kcal (<550) expenditure reduces risk - Type of activity not important	- Reduces risk of CAD by 20-30% if active - Greater activity levels lead to less CHF, fewer strokes, and lower mortality with fewer complications
T2DM Prevention	150 min/wk of moderate intensity	31% decreased risk of T2DM excluding BMI 17% decreased risk of T2DM including BMI Lowers HbA1c ONLY when dietary advice is added to exercise advice
Cancer Prevention	180-240 min/wk of mod-vig intensity; Dose-response relationship	20-30% decreased risk for breast cancer, risk of recurrence and mortality 17-30% decreased risk for colon cancer
Cancer Treatment	Any	Improves survival, quality of life, fitness
Disability	As active as possible	- Improve disability, mortality and maintain independence longer - May have mobility limitations, would benefit from expert assistance for safety
Weight Management	• >250 min/wk physical activity • 420 min/wk of exercise (moderate intensity) Strength training 2x/wk	- Need BOTH decreased calories and exercise, exercise alone can help, but requires a MUCH higher dose (e.g., A 1-mile walk/run burns only 100 calories) - Compensation: A study showed that if an overweight patient loses 1500 calories via exercise, he/she is likely to then consume 1000 additional calories, greatly reducing any weight-loss effect of exercise - National Weight Control Registry is the largest online registry of successful weight loss patients - Average patient did 420 min/wk exercise, lost 66 lbs, and kept it off for five years

Table 8-8. Physical Activity Guidelines for Americans 2018 – designed to provide guidance for physical activity recommendations to lead a healthy lifestyle

Age/ Condition	Aerobic Exercise	Resistance/ Strength	Flexibility	Comments
3-5 years	Active unstructured play	NONE		Adult assistance for encouragement
6-17 years	420 min/wk of mod-vigorous, with vigorous at least 3x/wk	60 min 3x/wk (e.g. tug of war, climbing, etc.)		Supervision advised if using weights
18-64 years	150-300 min/wk of moderate or 75-150 min/wk of vigorous	2-3 x/wk (non-consecutive days) of one set (8-12 reps) for each major muscle group	10 min 2-3x/wk; Goal is to hold each stretch 10-30 sec, 2-3x to get 60 sec/muscle	Can double amount of time spent in aerobic activity for additional benefits. Flexibility is best if performed daily

Specific balance exercises not necessarily needed for healthy kids and adults but is optional. Example: Standing on one leg first with hand support, then without hand support, then on an unstable surface such as foam board or bosu ball.

Table 8-9. Progression Guidelines from American College of Sports Medicine

Stage	Duration	What To Do
Initial	1-6 weeks	- 15 min, then go to 30 min - 3-4x/wk - Moderate intensity
Improvement	4-8 months	- 25-40 min - 3-5x/wk - Increase max HR by no more than 5% every 6 sessions
Maintenance	24+ weeks	- 20-60 min - 3-5x/wk - 70-85% of HRR

Table 8-10. Screening and Clearing Before Exercise:
Note: PAR-Q+ = The Physical Activity Readiness Questionnaire for Everyone

Who to screen?	Everyone, preferably using a self-administered tool called PAR-Q+
Who needs to be cleared before exercising?	**All symptomatic (see next line), all moderate/vigorous intensity in cardiac, metabolic, or renal disease**; no inherent need to clear light intensity or people w/ pulmonary disease
What is symptomatic?	ischemic discomfort, dizziness, orthopnea/paroxysmal nocturnal dyspnea, ankle edema, arrythmia, intermittent claudication, heart murmur, shortness of breath at rest or with mild activity
How to clear?	Stress test*
Why important?	Reduces exercise-related ACS events

Absolute contraindications: MI in <3 days, HTN emergency, acute myo/peri/endo-carditis, unstable angina, symptomatic heart failure, symptomatic severe aortic stenosis, uncontrolled arrythmia, acute PE, severe pulm HTN, or acute aortic dissection. Relative contraindications: high grade AV blocks, severe HTN >200mmHG / >110mmHg, inability to exercise due to physical/mental impairments, L main coronary stenosis, mod stenotic valvular heart disease, electrolyte abnormalities, tachy- or brady- arrhythmias, and hypertrophic cardiomyopathy

Figure 8-1. Who To Screen

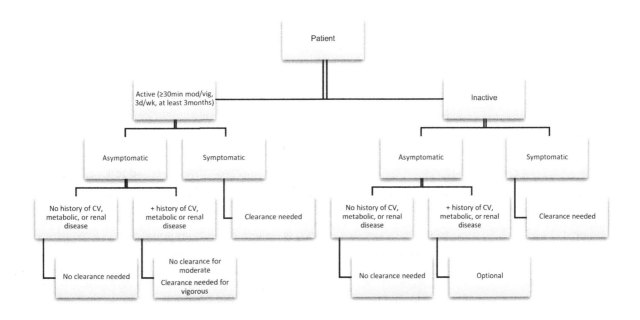

Table 8-11. Exercise Intensity

	Light	Moderate	Vigorous
METs	<3	3-5.9	>6
Talk test	Can talk and sing	Can talk, but not sing	Can barely talk
Maximal Heart Rate (MHR) *(220 - age)*	63% or less of max	64-76% of max	77-100% of max
Respiratory rate *(breaths/minute) (can use respiratory wearables)*	65% of respiration max	70% of respiration max	>80% of respiration max
Borg scale of perceived exertion (6-20 scale) *(Calculation from max HR/10)*	<12	12-13	>14
Borg category - ratio score (shortened version, 0-10)	<4	5-6	>7
Heart Rate Reserve *(MHR - resting HR)*X + resting HR*	X <40%	X = 40-59%	X ≥60%
Steps		3000 steps/30min	4000 steps/30min

Table 8-12. Components of Physical Fitness and Testing

Name of Test	What is Assessed?	How Test is Conducted
6-minute walk test*	Cardiorespiratory Fitness	Walk as far as you can in six minutes. Measure of ability to do Activities of Daily Living (ADLs) for older patients. More useful for tracking progress.
VO₂ max	Cardiorespiratory Fitness	Wear a mask and heart rate monitor while on treadmill or bike. The mask is connected to a machine that measures the volume of oxygen inhaled and the amount exhaled.
Step test	Cardiorespiratory Fitness	Take 12-inch steps for 3 minutes and then rest for 1 minute before HR measured and compared to norms for age/sex. Validated. Good for non-fit pts.
Submaximal talk test	Cardiorespiratory Fitness	Complex test requiring continuous telemetry.
Rockport fitness walking test	Cardiorespiratory Fitness	Walk one mile as fast as possible, then check HR. VO₂ is estimated with an equation.
Muscle strength	Muscle Strength	One-rep max with weights. Increase weight until muscle fatigue induced in 1-2 reps.
Grip strength	Muscle Strength	Can be used to predict mortality and function especially in older patients.
Vertical jump/ <10lb ball throw	Muscle Strength	Measuring maximum height / distance for jump / throw, used in athletes
8-Foot Up and Go	Muscle Strength	Sit to stand, walk 8 ft, circle a cone, walk back, sit; used in older adults to measure core body strength
Endurance	Muscular Endurance	Maximum number of correctly performed, consecutive repetitions (squats, sit-ups, etc.). Compare to age/sex norms.
Sit and reach test	Flexibility	Sit with heels touching box and reach as far as possible without bending knees; measure distance. Three chances given. Tests: hamstring flexibility moderately, but poor for low back flexibility.
Calipers	Body Composition	Measure skin fold (as ⅓ of body fat is subcutaneous, estimates body fat) at 3-7 sites. Optimal range (ACSM): Male = 10-22% Female = 20-32%
Bioimpedence	Body Composition	Electric current passing from one end to another; recently become more reliable
Densitometry (Gold standard)	Body Composition	DEXA scan or Hydrodensitometry (underwater weighing).
Short Performance Battery	Mobility *(Improvements here decrease long-term physical disability)*	**B**alance, **C**hair rise test, **G**ait speed test.

Similar absolute and relative contraindications to stress testing, but cut-offs are even lower.

Table 8-13. MET

Exercise Level	METs	Examples
Light	<3 METs	writing (1.5)
		walking slowly (2.0)
Moderate	3-6 METs	walking @ 3 mph (3.0)
		light housework (3.5)
		tennis (5.0)
		moderate weightlifting (5.0)
Vigorous	>6 METs	aerobic dance (6.0)
		bicycling @ 10-12 mph (6.0)
		basketball (8.0)
		jogging @ 6 mph (9.0)
		rope jumping (11.0)

METs are absolute, but as a person becomes more fit, she/he accomplishes more with less oxygen consumption, so these classifications may not be appropriate

Table 8-14. Minimum and Maximum Amounts of Exercise

MINIMUM	*There is no minimum amount of physical activity; any activity is helpful*	
Most Benefits	10-20 MET hours/wk	
Non-exercise	Benefits seen with fidgeting, standing, taking steps, etc.	
HIIT (high intensity interval training)	Brief vigorous activity with periods of rest or low-intensity activity may be good for fit individuals with time constraints, but more research needed	
MAXIMUM		
Benefit plateau	80 MET hours/wk	
Smaller additional risk reduction	Going past 150 minutes of moderate (or 75 minutes of vigorous) exercise yields much smaller incremental improvements in risk reduction or years of life gained:	
	- 4 MET hours/wk	2 years of life gained
	- 10 MET hours/wk	3 years of life gained
	- 22 MET hours/wk	4 years of life gained
Vigorous only	Vigorous exercise yields greater benefits than moderate exercise (five hours of life gained per 1 hr vs 2.6 hours of life per 1 hr of moderate)	

MET hours equals MET level (Table 8-9) multiplied by the number of hours (ex. 4 MET activity for 60min = 240min =4 MET hours)
(Source: Reimers CD et al. (2012) J Aging Res. 10.1155/2012/243958)

Table 8-15. Components of an Exercise Prescription

F	Frequency	Days/week
I	Intensity	Perceived exertion rating
T	Time	Minutes/session
T	Type	What was the exercise?
V	Volume	Amount of exercise/week
P	Progression	How to increase exercise intensity and/or duration

Table 8-16. Supporting Studies

Name of Study	Method	Result
Shanghai Women's Health Study	Studied 40-70-yr-old healthy but sedentary women, 1/2 of whom exercised regularly, while other 1/2 performed non-exercise physical activity.	- 20-40% risk reduction for all causes of mortality among the most active members of each group: - Women who walked >1 mile/day had hazard ratio of 0.65 - Women performing ≥4 of non-exercise physical activity had a hazard ratio of 0.60
Nurse's Health Study		- As little as 1-2 hr/wk of moderate to vigorous activity had significant reduction for all causes of mortality - Exercise above 7 hr/wk showed negligible incremental benefit
Activity Counseling Trial (ACT) Research Group	54 doctors received 3-4 min of exercise advice to give to sedentary patients	- 99% of patients got the advice - 86% of doctors spent less than 6 min - 83% of doctors thought it was helpful - 63% of doctors said no inc visit time - 46% of doctors spent 3-4 minutes
"Effectiveness of Physical Activity Advice and Prescription by Physicians in Routine Primary Care: A Cluster Randomized Trial" (Grandes 2009)	56 doctors counseled all patients; six months later, exercise activity was assessed	- Activity increased by 18 min in intervention group - Advice helped a little with adults >50 yrs old, but not at all with younger adults
	30% (a subgroup) also were given an exercise prescription	- Adults >50 yrs old inc activity by 131 min/wk and doubled their mod-vig activity - Adults <50 yrs old inc activity by 31.5 min/wk and had a 7% higher chance of meeting guidelines
		26 patients needed to get one sedentary person to meet activity guidelines.
Effectiveness of PA Promotion Based in Primary Care: Review of RCTs (Orrow 2012)	13 papers on physical activity counseling were reviewed	Counseling by primary care doctors does have a small-to-medium positive intervention effect at 12 months
		12 patients needed to treat to get one to meet physical activity guidelines at one year (vs. 50-120 to stop smoking).

Table 8-17. Additional Resources

Topic	Resource	Comments
Self-monitoring	Pedometer, Fitbit or other wearable, phone alarm, partner, app, etc.	
Health Promotion Clinic	Brief physical activity counseling by PCP led to 31% increase in patients remembering to exercise*	
Team Members	Physical Therapist	Limited number of visits covered, usually related to injury or surgery.
	Exercise Physiologist	Supervises exercise, but not usually covered by insurance.
	Fitness/Wellness/Health Coach	Can be expensive, not covered by insurance, and much variability in experience.
	Personal Trainer	Not covered by insurance, variable experience and knowledge
Wellness Programs	Examples include: - Walk with a Doc - Let's Move - Silver Sneakers - The President's Challenge - Exercise is Medicine - Team incentives with tracking	
Worksite Wellness Programs	Motorola's wellness program**	For every $1 spent, ROI was $3.93 (Total: $6.5 million) Participating employees spent 2.5% more on health costs, compared to 18% for non-participants.
	Other typical programs	For every $1 spent, return on investment was $3.
Other resources	Gyms, health clubs, 5K events, parks, etc.	

*Lobelo F, Duperly J, Frank E. Physical activity habits of doctors and medical students influence their counselling practices. *British Journal of Sports Medicine* 2009;**43**:89-92. *http://dx.doi.org/10.1136/bjsm.2008.055426*
***Jnl Workplace Beh Health 2005; 20(3-4):203-218. https://doi.org/10.1300/J490v20n03_01*

Table 8-18. Physical Activity Team Members

Team Member	Focus	Cost/Insurance
Physical Therapist	Restore function and reduce pain	$$ / Limited #/year
Occupational Therapist	Activities of Daily Living	$$ / Limited #/year
Clinical Exercise Physiologists (bachelor's/master's in exercise)	Designing and carrying out an exercise rx/plan	$$$ / not covered
Coaches – varying certifications	Fitness, wellness, or health	$$ / not covered
Certified Personal Trainers – 18 accrediting bodies	Fitness assessment, setting goals, and carrying out a plan	$$$ / not covered

CHAPTER 9
SLEEP HEALTH

Definitions

Chronotype: The body's natural inclination to sleep at a certain time, genetically linked ("morning lark" or "night owl")

Circadian rhythm: The natural cycle and synchronization of physical, mental, and behavioral changes that the body goes through during one day ("body clock")

Entrainment: The ability to be brought into (circadian) rhythm by external factors

Glymphatic system: Increased "flushing" of the brain by CSF during sleep ("waste removal") - akin to the body's lymphatic system

Sleep propensity: The ability to transition to sleep when awake and to stay asleep

Sleep (onset) latency: The time to transition from fully awake to asleep

Sleep efficiency: Equals time asleep divided by time in bed

Table 9-1. Association of Inadequate or Poor Sleep with Chronic Disease Pathophysiology

	Changes with Inadequate or Poor Sleep	Chronic Disease Associations
Immune	- Decreased antibody production - Increased inflammatory mediators - Epigenetic changes	Frequent viral or bacterial infections, autoimmune disorders
Metabolic	- Increased cortisol levels - Increased blood glucose - Decreased growth hormone - Disturbance of gut microbiome - Epigenetic changes	Overweight/obesity, insulin resistance, prediabetes, T2DM, metabolic syndrome
Cardiovascular	- Increased sympathetic tone - Increased vasospasm - Increased AGE (advanced glycation end product) deposition in vasculature - Increased endothelial dysfunction	Hypertension, acute myocardial infarction, fatal coronary events, vasospastic disorders, dyslipidemia
Mental Health	- Impaired memory/processing - Decreased fear extinguishment - Impaired moral judgement - Decreased concentration/alertness	Major depressive disorder, bipolar, seasonal affective disorder, PMS, PTSD, Alzheimer's disease
Cancer	- Decreased DNA repair - Aberrant DNA methylation	Breast, endometrial, prostate, colorectal cancers
Reproductive	- Decreased testosterone - Decreased sperm quality and count - Decreased FSH (follicular stimulating hormone)	Infertility

Table 9-2. Sleep Disorders

	Symptoms	Effects	At-Risk Populations
Behaviorally Induced Insufficient Sleep Syndrome *(also called "social jet lag")*	Voluntary sleep restriction, longer sleep times on weekends	Inadequate sleep for quality performance *(Presenteeism: Present but not productive at work)*	30s, work week >40 hrs, increased stress, increased alcohol use, depression
Insomnia	Difficulty initiating or maintaining sleep despite adequate opportunity >three months duration and at least 3x/wk	Daytime consequences include: - Fatigue - Memory/concentration impairment - Decreased motivation - Mood disturbance - Work/car accidents - Anxiety about sleep - Physical symptoms (headache, GI)	

Obstructive Sleep Apnea	- Recurrent apnea (cessation of breathing) or hypopnea (shallow breathing) associated with arousals
	- Diagnosed on PSG
	- AHI 5-15 (mild)
	  AHI 15-30 (moderate)
	  AHI 30+ (severe)
		- Daytime fatigue
		- Morning headaches
		- Work/car accidents
		- In children, enuresis, behavioral issues
			- Overweight/obese
			- Metabolic syndrome
			- HTN
			- Atrial fibrillation
			- Large neck circumference
			- Loud snoring

Narcolepsy	- Sudden, uncontrollable sleep onset - From awake directly into REM (skip NREM)	- With or without cataplexy (sudden loss of muscle tone while awake, often triggered by a sudden, strong emotion) - Diagnosis of exclusion (need PSG to rule out other causes)	- Slightly more common in men - Symptoms usually start during teen years
Shift Work Sleep Disorder	Due to shift work (nights, rotating shifts)	May cause secondary insomnia and drowsiness at work	Listed as probable carcinogen (Group 2A) by WHO

Table 9-2 (cont.). Sleep Disorders

	Symptoms	Effects	Demographics
Periodic Limb Movements	- Limb movements causing brief arousals, but patient unaware - Seen on PSG	- Often associated with Restless Leg Syndrome (RLS), but not the same - May complain of daytime sleepiness	Increases with age, especially over 50 years old
Restless Leg Syndrome (RLS)	Sensorimotor disorder with the urge to move legs due to uncomfortable feeling (paresthesia, pain) when sitting or lying down; worse in evenings	- Periodic limb movements while sleeping in 85% - Phase delay and sleep disruptions - Daytime fatigue - Periodic involuntary/jerky limb movements when awake	- Can be genetic or acquired - Can have low ferritin (<75 ng/ml) or elevated ferritin - Magnesium deficient (doesn't correlate with serum measurement) - Vitamin D deficient
REM Sleep Behavior Disorder	Vocalizations or aggressive movements during REM phase		Older patients with neurodegenerative diseases
Short Sleep Misperception	Mismatch between sleep duration (PSG) and patient reported sleep time		
Secondary Insomnia	Due to medication, vascular disease, visual impairment, abnormality of renin-angiotensin system		

Table 9-3. Sleep Recommendations, by Age

Age	Amount of Sleep Recommended *(hours per day)*
Newborn (0-3 months)	14-17
4-12 months	12-16 *(including naps)*
1-2 years	11-14 *(including naps)*
3-5 years	10-13 *(including naps)*
6-12 years	9-12
12-18 years	8-10
Adults (19-64 years)	7-9
Seniors (65+ years)	7-8

Table 9-4. Sleep Phase Shift

Phase Delay *(body is delayed compared to time clock)*	Phase Advance *(body is ahead of time clock)*
Sleep onset and awakening delayed (compared to solar cycle) *Evening light (residential 100-1000 lux) can delay sleep onset by 1-3 hrs and can cause almost 100% melatonin suppression*	Premature sleep onset and awakening (compared to solar cycle)
Eastward travel across time zones *Remaining awake even though the clock shows it is bedtime and/or it is dark outside ("delayed" or "behind the clock")*	Westward travel* across time zones *Feeling sleepy despite it being light outside ("advanced" or "ahead of the clock")*
Night owl	Morning lark
Spring: Daylight saving time change *(clock advances, leaving body in a "delayed" state)*	Fall: Daylight saving time change *(clock moves back; body now "ahead" of it)*
Treatment: - Expose to bright light upon awakening - Eat high calorie breakfast within 30-45 min of ideal wakeup time - Increase morning physical activity - Get only dim light exposure starting 1 hr before new bedtime - 1 mg melatonin 1 hr before new bedtime	Treatment: - Delay bright light exposure upon awakening until closer to ideal time - Eat high calorie breakfast/have caffeine 30-45 min after ideal wakeup time - Increase bright light exposure in evening - Increase evening physical activity - Eat complex carb rich dinner 2-3 hrs before new bedtime - Avoid dim light at night until 1 hr before new bedtime - 1 mg melatonin 1 hr before new bedtime

Suprachiasmatic nucleus can only adjust by one hour per day in new time zone

Table 9-5. General Sleep Assessment

	Topic	Scale	Abnormal	Recommend-ation
History of Present Illness (HPI) questions	Sleep patterns	-Typical hours -Typical bedtime/ wake time - Perceived quality - Daytime tiredness - Sleep latency >15-20 min - Attitude	Red flags: - <7 hrs or >9 hrs - >1 hr difference in duration between week/wknd - >1 hr difference in bed/wake times - night shift work or irregular shifts - self-reported poor quality	PSQI or MSQ
Pittsburgh Sleep Quality Index (PSQI)	Sleep quality and patterns	- 19 items, 0-3 scale - seven component scores - answers reflect past month	>5 indicates poor sleeper Components: subjective sleep quality, duration, latency, efficiency, disturbances, use of sleeping meds, daytime dysfunction	Further screening
Mini Sleep Assessment (MSQ)	Sleep quality and excessive daytime somnolence (EDS)	- 10 questions - 7 point Likert scale - 2 sub-scales: daytime sleepiness and sleep quality	Scoring: 10-24 good 25-27 mild sleep problem 28-30 moderate problem >30 severe sleep problem	Further screening
Actigraphy	Movements recorded over time	-Wearables (Fitbit, Smart watches) not validated -More accurate than sleep log, but less than PSG	More accurate for sleep duration	PSQI or MSQ

Table 9-6. Lifestyle Interventions That Can Improve Sleep Health

Topic	Factors	Interventions
Light Exposure	Amount	Pupil Size, Sunglasses, Cataracts
	Timing	Low daytime light increases susceptibility to melatonin suppression from bright evening/night light, even at residential lighting intensity (100-150 lux)
		Bright light therapy: 10,000 lux 20-30 min upon awakening
		Increase midday light exposure (preferably outside) Noon sunlight ~100K lux
		Decrease light exposure about 1 hr prior to bedtime (dim lights/use lamps)
	Color	Short wavelengths (blue/green) suppress melatonin more than high intensity long wavelength (red) light
		Blue light blockers for screens
		Avoid electronics/blue light 1-2 hrs before bedtime
	Frequency	One day of irregular light exposure can affect melatonin levels for the next 2-3 nights
	Temperature	Use 2500K light temperature in home (warm and soft)
Temperature	External	Ideal thermostat setting is 65-67°F
	Core body temp cooling/cutaneous warming	Enhance core body cooling with sauna, warm bath/shower, socks, yoga 1-2 hours before bed
Fluids	Dehydration	Increased blood osmolality → increased antidiuretic hormone (ADH) → increased water resorption → increased vascular tone → increased cardiac output to muscles → increased core body temperature (CBT)
		Maintain steady hydration throughout the day, loading earlier in the morning and tapering later in evening to avoid late night bathroom trips
	Diuretics	Avoid caffeine, alcohol, soda in afternoon/evening
	Sodium	Avoid high salt intake, especially in evening
		Increased vascular volume → increased urine output overnight

Table 9-6 (cont.). Lifestyle Interventions That Can Improve Sleep Health

Food	Breakfast	Don't skip breakfast, may aid in AM cortisol peak and sync you with circadian rhythm
	Dinner	Avoid dinner rich in simple carbs/sugar, may delay sleep onset by increasing insulin/cortisol response
	Timing	Dinner should be >3 hrs prior to bed to decrease reflux and avoid rise in CBT Eliminate after dinner/bedtime/middle-of-night snacks If evening snack is necessary, choose small serving of protein-rich item
Exercise	AM/early afternoon	Advances sleep phase (makes you feel sleepy earlier), good for patients struggling with sleep latency Increase early AM and afternoon activity, but don't overdo it (pain can disrupt sleep)
	Evening	Delays phase (makes you feel sleepy later), good for patients who have trouble staying asleep Exercise >2 hrs prior to bedtime to avoid CBT elevation that could interfere
Substances	Alcohol	Avoid completely or limit to early evening intake (>3 hrs before bedtime, less than 2 drinks) Causes sedation (vs. good quality sleep); decreases REM phase, increases sleep fragmentation, inhibits ADH therefore acts as diuretic increasing urine output overnight
	Caffeine	Limit daytime caffeine and try to avoid after 2pm Reduces sleepiness (adenosine blocker), reduces Stage 3 sleep (deep sleep)
Stress reduction		Start a bedtime or wind-down routine about 1 hr prior to bedtime Incorporate active relaxation: bath, soft music, meditation, mindfulness-based stress reduction (MBSR)

Table 9-7. Sleep Assessments for OSA, Insomnia, and Restless Leg Syndrome

	Topic	Scale	Abnormal	Recommendation
Epworth Sleep Scale (ESS)	Daytime sleepiness	- Eight situations - Likelihood of falling sleep on a scale of 0 (never) to 3 (often)	>eight abnormal Situations: sitting reading, watching TV, inactive in public place, car passenger >1 hr, lying down in afternoon, sitting and talking, sitting after lunch, in car stopped in traffic	Sleep study if abnormal, consider referral to sleep specialist
STOP-BANG	Sleep Apnea	Eight factors: **S**noring, **T**ired, **O**bserved Apnea, Blood **P**ressure, **B**MI >35, **A**ge >50, **N**eck size (≥17in M, ≥16in F), **G**ender	0-2 low risk 3-4 interim risk 5-8 high risk But also **high** risk if 2 of the STOP questions and 1 of these BANG issues: - BMI - Neck - Male	Sleep study for high risk, consider referral to sleep specialist
Insomnia Severity Index (ISI)	Insomnia	7 questions rated 0-4 by severity	0-7 -No clinically significant insomnia 8-14 -Subthreshold insomnia 15-21 -Clinical insomnia (moderate severity) 22-28 - Clinical insomnia (severe)	Sleep hygiene, CBTi, consider referral to sleep specialist
Restless Leg Syndrome Questionnaire (RLSQ)	Restless Leg Syndrome	10 questions rated 0-4 by severity	0 None 1-10 Mild 11-20 Moderate 21-30 Severe 31-40 Very severe	Consider referral to specialist for RLS treatment

Table 9-8. CBT* (Cognitive Behavioral Therapy for Insomnia)

Cognitive restructuring	Addressing anxiety or erroneous beliefs about sleep	See Table 3-17 for CBT methods
Behavioral *(only sleep restriction and stimulus control proven effective for adults >60 years)*	Sleep restriction	1. Restrict time in bed 2. Set strict wakeup time based on logged *sleep* time in past 3. Gradually increase time in bed AND asleep 4. Aim for sleep efficiency >80%
	Stimulus control	Strengthen bed as cue for sleep (e.g. read in a different dimly lit room until groggy)
	Relaxation training	Guided imagery of relaxing muscle groups
Sleep hygiene		See Table 9-6

*1st line treatment for insomnia

CHAPTER 10
MANAGING TOBACCO CESSATION AND RISKY ALCOHOL USE

Tobacco Use

Table 10-1. How Cigarettes Have Changed

Changes to:	Results Compared to 1970
Filters	New filters with ventilation holes cause smokers to inhale more frequently and vigorously
Additives	Higher levels of 70 carcinogens (includes bronchodilators and cough suppressants)
Addiction potential	10-25% of smokers will develop symptoms of addiction after only 1 cig
Cancer potential	Smokers more likely to develop lung adenocarcinoma than in past

https://www.tobaccofreekids.org › press-releases › 2014. doi: 10.1006/pmed.1997.0212

Table 10-2. Smoking and Medical Conditions

Deaths from Smoking	Illnesses Worsened by Smoking
#1 cause of preventable morbidity and mortality in US *(Smoking causes ½ million deaths/yr)*	Diabetes (smokers have increased risk of DM by 35%)
87% of lung cancer deaths	Rheumatoid arthritis
80% of deaths from COPD	Tuberculosis
50% of all smokers will die as a result of smoke related illness	Immune system functioning
33% of all cancer deaths (acute myeloid leukemia, bladder, lung, cervix, colorectal, esophagus, kidney, liver, oral cavity and pharynx, pancreas, stomach, and larynx	Cancer treatment failure rate
32% of coronary heart disease deaths	Pregnancy complications, including ectopic pregnancy, preterm delivery, stillbirth
20% of all U.S. deaths	Newborn complications, including low birth weight, SIDS, cleft lip and palate
	Age-related macular degeneration
	Erectile dysfunction
	Reproductive disability in both men and women
	Poor wound healing
	Muscle pains

Table 10-3. Benefits of Quitting Smoking

Timeframe	Benefit
Immediate	Cut risk of heart attack by 50% of those who still smoke
Minutes	Heart rate and blood pressure decrease
1 day	Nicotine level drops to 0
1-2 months	Cough and shortness of breath decreases
1 year	Cut risk of heart disease by 50%
2-5 years	Risk of stroke is same as non-smoker
10 years	Cuts risk of lung cancer by 50%
15 years	Risk of coronary heart disease close to non-smoker
20 years	Risk of oral cancer and pancreatic cancer close to non-smoker
Quit at age 30	Gain 10 years of life
Quit at age 60	Gain 3 years of life
Quit any time	Better quality of life, less disability, less respiratory, cardiovascular disease including strokes and aneurysms

Table 10-4. How Five A's of Tobacco Cessation Differ from Behavior Change Model

Tobacco Cessation	Behavior Change
Ask: All patients should be asked if they smoke	**Assess:** Personalize health risk
Advise: SMART rx	**Advise**
Assess: Is patient ready to make a quit attempt?	**Agree:** What should we focus on and is patient ready?
Assist	**Assist**
Arrange	**Arrange**

See Health Behavior Change chapter 3 for counseling techniques

Table 10-5. Counseling Methods and Effectiveness

Method	How It's Done	Effectiveness
Stopping on one's own	Patient does it by herself/himself	- 5% effective overall - 50% resume within 14 days - 75% resume within 30 days
Doctor's guidance	- Brief (<3 mins) discussion - Personal, group (more intense and especially if in person; >4 sessions is best) - Telephone quit lines (very effective) - Behavioral therapy - Intensive person-to-person contact - Medications are encouraged; counseling and meds (most effective) - All should include problem solving for triggers, building coping skills, social support, and use of multiple formats for best results.	- Success rate doubled compared to doing by herself/himself - 40-50% stop by three months

Note: Relapse is a normal part of the process! If patient is not ready, use motivational Interviewing

Table 10-6(a). Medications to Help Quit Smoking: Standard Single Therapies
(Note: 14% of Americans still smoke)

Rank	Therapy	Action	Effectiveness	Comments
—	Placebo	None	- 30% stopped at two months - 21% stopped at three months - 17% stopped at six months	Nicotine is the most common chemical dependence in US
1st line	Nicotine patch	Nicotine replacement therapies (NRT): Stimulates nicotinic receptors in ventral tegmental area leading to dopamine release	45% stopped at two months	OTC
	Nicotine gum		40% stopped at 2 months	OTC
	Nicotine lozenge		40% stopped at 2 months	OTC
	Nicotine inhaler		Decreased consumption by 50% at 4 months	Prescription
	Nicotine nasal spray		Decreased consumption by 50% at 4 months	Prescription
	Varenicline	Nicotinic receptor PARTIAL agonist	- 51% stopped at 3 months - 35% stopped at 6 months	Most effective monotherapy: Prevents withdrawals and stops nicotine highs
	Bupropion	Inhibits reuptake of both norepi and dopamine	40% stopped at 2 months	
2nd line	Clonidine	Acts on the CNS to reduce withdrawal symptoms	Case-by-case basis	Only use if first line meds not effective or not indicated
	Nortriptyline	Unclear mechanism, but thought to be related to lower dopamine activity reducing the rewards of smoking	Case-by-case basis	Only use if first line meds not effective or not indicated

Table 10-6(b). Medications to Help Quit Smoking: Other Treatment Options

Type	Treatment	Effectiveness	Comments
Combos	Varenicline + Bupropion	71% stopped at three months 58% stopped at six months	**Most effective treatment**
	Bupropion + Nicotine Replacement (1-2)	35-54% stopped at two months	Mental health/chronic disease
Alternatives	Acupuncture	Insufficient effective	E-cigarettes: · Not FDA controlled, inconsistent ingredients · Can be poisonous if swallowed or absorbed through skin or mucous membranes · May be contaminated with heavy metals or carcinogens · EVALI (**E**-cigarette/**VA**ping **L**ung **I**njury) can be serious and caused by vitamin E acetate in vape material
	Hypnosis	Insufficient effective	
	Biofeedback	Insufficient evidence	
	Cigarette fading	Insufficient evidence	
	Incentives	Insufficient evidence	
	E-cigarettes, vaping, e-hookah	Insufficient evidence; most adults continue to use BOTH e-cigarettes and cigarettes	

Table 10-7. Smoking and Special Populations

Patient Type	Comments
Teenagers	10.5% and 27.6% are using e-cigarettes in middle and high school, respectively; Nicotine harms growing brains; treatment options: educational programs, NRT>>smoking.
Cancer patients	Higher cancer treatment failure rate.
Pregnant patients*	Counseling is best but can use **OTC** replacement treatment if needed. However, do NOT use prescription replacement treatment, as this can cause birth defects. Also, Bupropion and Varenicline are Category C risk.
Light smokers (<10 cig/day)	CBT; NRT is not shown to be beneficial
Smokeless tobacco users	CBT
Chronic disease patients	Triple medication (Bupropion, patch, and one nicotine replacement treatment) recommended
Cardiovascular patients	- No increase in MI if on patch and still smoke - Nicotine replacement treatment advises caution if acute disease present
Comorbid Mental Health Disorder	- Most will need medication, may need higher doses, longer duration, and often combo treatment - For bipolar, NO Bupropion; use only patch - For schizophrenia, use patch

Notes: 1. There is insufficient evidence for almost all of these special populations because of high risk of studies on these populations. Much of these recs are based on best judgment. 2. NRT = Nicotine Replacement Therapy

*PREGNANCY AND SMOKING CESSATION TREATMENTS

For pregnant women who are not able to quit successfully with behavioral therapy alone:
- Short-acting oral nicotine replacement therapy (NRT) ad lib.
- Nicotine patch in lowest effective dose if oral NRT is ineffective
- Combination NRT, if needed
- Bupropion alone or added to NRT, if needed
- No data on varenicline safety

(Source: https://www.mayo.edu/research/documents/ndep-082013a-tobacco-dependence-treatment-pregnancy-pdf/doc-20012880)

The 10 Most Important Recommendations from the U.S. Public Health Service

1. Tobacco dependence is a Chronic Disease for which effective treatments exist, but often requires repeated attempts and close follow-up.
2. Physicians should always document and ask about tobacco use.
3. There are effective treatments for all who want to change.
4. Brief interventions lasting less than three minutes will increase abstinence.
5. More intense treatment is more effective in a dose response manner, with more than four in-person sessions that include problem-solving and skills training and have social support being most effective.
6. Medication, especially combo treatment, should be encouraged if not contraindicated.
7. Medication and counseling together is better than either method alone.
8. Patients should be given access to telephone "quitline" counseling.
9. Use motivational interviewing if patient is not ready to quit.
10. Treatment for tobacco dependence is particularly cost effective.

Table 10.8. Insurance Coverage for Smoking Cessation

Program	Coverage
Medicare *(mainly age 65+)*	- Cessation meds: nicotine nasal spray, nicotine inhaler, bupropion and varenicline. *(Part D plans may opt to cover other meds.)* - 4 sessions of individual counseling for up to 2 quit attempts/yr - No cost-sharing for counseling or annual prevention visit
Medicaid *(usually low income or disabilities)*	- *For pregnant women:* Individual, group, and phone counseling; all FDA-approved smoking cessation meds - *For all Medicaid enrollees:* All FDA-approved smoking cessation medications

Medicaid Expansion	- *Federal guidance defines "preventative services" as:*
	  o 4 sessions of individual, group and phone counseling.
	  o 90 days of all FDA-approved smoking cessation meds
	  o 2 quit attempts per year.
	  o No prior authorization for treatments and no cost-sharing

State Health Insurance *(usually earnings of 100-400% of poverty level)*	- Same as Federal guidelines for preventative services, as described above
Employer-Sponsored Plan	- Same as Federal guidelines for preventative services, as described above

Table 10-9. Lung Cancer Screening, Ages 50-80 (USPSTF)

Smoking History	Still Smoking? / Other Factors	What to Do
20 pack-years	Yes	Annual LDCT scan
20 pack-years	No; quit ≤ 15 years ago	Annual LDCT scan
20 pack-years	No; quit > 15 years ago	None
20 pack-years	Serious health issue or wouldn't consider curative lung surgery	None

NOTE: Screening high-risk persons with low-dose CT screening (LDCT) can reduce lung cancer mortality and may reduce all-cause mortality but can also yield false-positive results through unnecessary tests and procedures, overdiagnosis, incidental findings, increases in distress, and, rarely, radiation-induced cancers. (Source: US Preventative Services Task Force)

Alcohol Use

Table 10-10. Incidence of AUD (Alcohol Use Disorder) in the United States

% of Adult Population:	Extent of Alcohol Use
30%	US adults exceed NIH guidelines at least 1x/yr
26%	US adults are "at risk" drinkers or have mild AUD
3%	US adults have moderate AUD
1%	US adults have severe AUD

Table 10-11. Populations at Higher Risk of AUD

Northeast, upper Midwest, Alaska, and Hawaii are more likely to binge
18-28 years old
Higher prevalence associated with higher income
Whites > Blacks
Men (23%) > Women (11%)
Smokers
Mental Illness
Patients who have had trauma
Family history of alcohol misuse

Screening Frequency: Screen **all** adults **annually** with "One Question" screen (USPSTF Grade B recommendation). If at higher risk, as in special populations noted above, or with clinical suspicion, may screen more frequently.

Table 10-12. Definition of a Drink

Definition of a Drink *(14g = 0.6 ounces pure alcohol)*		
Beverage	**Container Size**	**Drinks per Container**
Beer (5% alcohol/volume)	12 oz small can/bottle *(340g)*	1
	16 oz Pint/draft *(450g)*	1.3
Malt Liquor (~7% alc/vol) a higher alcohol beer made from malted barley	12 oz	1.5
	16 oz	2
Wine (12% alc/vol)	Glass 5 oz *(142g)*	1
	Bottle 25 oz *(750 ml)*	5
Hard Liquor/distilled spirits *(80 proof)* (40% alc/vol)	A "Shot" 1.5 oz *(34g)*	1
	Mixed drink/cocktail	1-1.5
	A "fifth" 25 oz *(750ml)*	17
	A liter *(34 oz)*	24

Table 10-13. Drinking Classification

Category of Drinking	Women	Men
Moderate	1 drink/day	2 drinks/day
At Risk (exceeds *daily mod level* **any** *day or* **any** *week;* **or** *binges at least 1x/month*)	2 drinks/day	3 drinks/day
Heavy (NIAAA)	>3 drinks/day or >7 drinks/wk	>4 drinks/day or >14 drinks/wk
Heavy (SAMHSA)	Binges >5 days/month	Binges >5 days/month
Binge (NIAAA) *(blood alcohol level of .08 mg/l)*	4 drinks (in 2 hours)	5 drinks (in 2 hours)
Binge (SAMHSA)	4 drinks (on same day) on at least 1 day in past month	5 drinks (on same day) on at least 1 day in past month

NIAAA = National Institute on Alcohol Abuse and Alcoholism
SAMHSA = Substance Abuse and Mental Health Services Administration

Table 10-14. Alcohol Screening

	Frequency	Scale	Abnormal	Recommendation
Alcohol screen	Annual screen	1 question: How many times have you had alcohol.	M: >4/d or 14/wk F: >3/day or 7/wk	Do an AUDIT
*AUDIT-C	If screen is positive, continue to follow	3 Q, 0-4 scale 1. days/wk 2. drinks/day 3. How often >6/d	M: >4 F: >3 Elderly M: >3	Identifies at risk, may need further screening
AUDIT 10	If screen is positive, continue to follow (**doesn't diagnose** AUD)	10 Q, 0-4	0-7 (low risk) 8-15 (mod risk) 16-19 (high risk) >20 (dependent)	Educate Brief intervention Brief int. With f/u Refer for treatment

C = consumption

CAGE Questionnaire (Johns Hopkins)

Can be used for problem drinking or drug use:

C. Have you ever felt you should **Cut** down on your drinking?
A. Have people **Annoyed** you by criticizing your drinking?
G. Have you ever felt bad or **Guilty** about your drinking?
E. Have you ever had a drink first thing in the morning to steady your nerves or to get rid of a hangover (**Eye-opener**)?

Score: Questions are scored 0 for "no" and 1 for "yes" answers, with a higher score being an indication of alcohol problems. A score of 2 or greater is considered clinically significant, although even 1 may be.

Table 10-14. Eleven DSM-5 Criteria-Based Questions to Determine (AUD)

"In the past year, have you ever....":	
1	… had times when you ended up drinking more, or longer, than you intended?
2	… more than once wanted to cut down or stop drinking, or tried to, but couldn't?
3	… spent a lot of time drinking? Or being sick or getting over other aftereffects?
4	… wanted a drink so badly you couldn't think of anything else?
5	… found that drinking—or being sick from drinking—often interfered with taking care of your home or family? Or caused job troubles? Or school problems?
6	… continued to drink even though it was causing trouble with your family or friends?
7	… given up or cut back on activities that were important or interesting to you, or gave you pleasure, in order to drink?
8	… more than once gotten into situations while or after drinking that increased your chances of getting hurt (such as driving, swimming, using machinery, walking in a dangerous area, or having unsafe sex)?
9	… continued to drink even though it was making you feel depressed or anxious or adding to another health problem? Or after having had a memory blackout?
10	… had to drink much more than you once did to get the effect you want? Or found that your usual number of drinks had much less effect than before?
11	… found that when the effects of alcohol were wearing off, you had withdrawal symptoms, such as trouble sleeping, shakiness, restlessness, nausea, sweating, a racing heart, or a seizure? Or sensed things that were not there?
Mild = 2-3 symptoms Moderate = 4-5 symptoms Severe = > 6 symptoms	

10-15. Anti-Relapse Medications for Alcohol Use Disorder
(can be prescribed by a non-specialist)

Medication	Helps with Heavy Drinking?	Reduces Drinking Days?	Treatment level
Naltrexone, 50 mg qd/bid *(blocks mu-opioid receptor)*	Yes; down by 83%	Yes; down by 4%	1st line
Acamprosate, 666 mg tid *(modulates glutamate neuro transmission)*	No	Yes; plus increased abstinence duration by 11 days	1st line *(Best used after drinking has stopped)*
Disulfiram, 250 mg qd *(inhibits aldehyde dehydrogenase)*	No	No	2nd line *(Bad side effects often leads to non-compliance)*
Gabapentin, 300 mg bid *(often much higher dose needed)*	No	Yes; by as much as 10-17%	2nd line *(Well-tolerated, but abuse potential)*
Topiramate, 100 mg bid	Yes; down by 43%	No	Off-label

Table 10-16 Treatment Stratified by AUD Classification

Diagnosis	Risks	Treatment
At risk/mild AUD	- AUD progression - Liver disease - Marital and family issues	- Brief counseling (up to 4 sessions) - Naltrexone prn - Follow-up - AAA support groups
Mild-moderate AUD	- AUD progression - Liver disease - Marital and family issues	- Primary care setting - Behavioral therapy (especially CBT) - Medications are equally as effective as counseling
Severe AUD *(often has prior risk factors)*	- Numerous life-threatening medical complications - Withdrawal symptoms can be severe	- Referral to addiction specialist - Family support, when appropriate - Anti-relapse meds, which help improve the number of patients who enter long term recovery

CHAPTER 11
EMOTIONAL HEALTH AND MENTAL WELL-BEING

Table 11-1 Useful Definitions

Term	Definition
Stress Reaction	Acting habitually or automatically irrespective of situational factors
Stress Response	Acting based on the situation in the moment, while maintaining awareness and acceptance of one's feelings
Allostatic Load	Cumulative burden of chronic stress and life events
Necessary Suffering	Unavoidable universal life experiences, including getting older, losing a loved one, and illnesses
Unnecessary Suffering	Self-inflicted based on egocentricity and our personal preferences. Suffering that is not 1 of the 3 necessary ones.
Formal Mindfulness	Dedicated time allotted to meditation
Informal Mindfulness	Awareness of moments occurring in everyday activities, reflecting on emotions and sensations more deeply Informal mindfulness creates distance between stimulus and a response, allowing for more processing and greater awareness in day-to-day life Attitudes: • Non-judging (witnessing) • Non-striving (relaxing) • Acknowledging • Patience • Self-reliance • Open-mindedness

Table 11-2. Non-Pharmacologic Stress and Depression Management Techniques

Address Lifestyle Factors (e.g. diet*, substances)	Formal Mindfulness Exercises (e.g. meditation)
Cardiorespiratory Exercise / Tai chi / Yoga**	Cognitive Behavior Therapy (CBT) or other therapy**
Massage	Spiritual/Religious Activity
Nature Immersion	Volunteering
Light Therapy: 10,000 lux for 30 min for SAD	Arts and Creativity
Learning Healthy Coping Skills	Lean on Social Support / Community
Maintaining mindful attitude (awareness, openness, patience, positivity, and not angling for anything)	

*Anti-depressive diet – less refined grains, sugar, and meat; more olive oil, vegetables, and fruit
**CBT + pharmacological therapies > Pharmacological therapies > exercise = CBT > no treatment. Less relapse of depression with CBT than with drugs.

Table 11-3. Mental Health Impact on Physical Health

Diabetes	- Bidirectionality of diabetes w/ depression: Diabetes predicts depression and depression predicts diabetes - Suicide ideation in people with diabetes increases if they have an A1c $\geq$6.5, are on insulin, or have had diabetes for $\geq$5 years
CAD	- CAD is associated with depression, and depression increases the risk of cardiac events - Depression is an independent marker for mortality as strong as tobacco use - Independent RF for cardiac events - Increases cardiac risk by 15-20% in people with CAD - Endothelial dysfunction - Lower heart rate variability - TCAs not recommended for ppl with CAD (bc of QT prolongation) - First line is SSRIs - Ideally, do meds + non-med therapies
Chronic Disease	- Depression/Stress is pro-inflammatory, leading to many chronic diseases - People with chronic diseases will often have a diagnosis of depression
Physical	- Stress prompts physical responses, like a clenched jaw or clenched fists

(Sources:
Lee H-Y, Hahm, M, Lee, S. Risk of suicidal ideation in diabetes varies by diabetes regimen, diabetes duration, and HbA1c level. J Psychosom Res. 2014; 76(4):275-9.
Jiang, Wei. Impacts of depression and emotional distress on cardiac disease. Cleveland Clinic Journal of Medicine March 2008, 75 (3 suppl 2) S20-S25.
Frasure-Smith, N, Lesperance, F. Depression and anxiety as predictors of 2-year cardiac events in patients with stable coronary disease. Arch Gen Psychiatry. 2008 Jan;65(1):62-71.)

10 categories of causes of poor mental health:
- Genetic
- Developmental – Adverse Childhood Experiences
- Physical activity
- Sleep
- Addiction
- Nutritional
- Toxic exposures
- Social stressors
- Medical - cancer, thyroid, diabetes (SI RFs are insulin therapy, duration of diabetes, and HbA1c >= 6.5), trauma, autoimmune, stroke
- Frontal lobe

SMILES study – 2018, 12 week RCT, parallel group, moderate to severe depression

- Vegetables (6 per day)
- Fruit (3 per day)

Diverse gut microbiome reduces the risk of depression.

Table 11-4. Screening Tools for Stress, Depression, and Anxiety

Satisfaction with Life Scale (SWLS)	Emotional Well-being	Higher age, levels of education, and income associated w/ greater well-being; "other" race (not white, black, or Hispanic), lowest level of education, and lower household income associated w/ lower well-being
Perceived Stress Scale Assessment	**Stress**	**Dr. Cohen; 1983; 10 items; 0-13 – low stress, 14-26 – mod stress, 27-40 – high stress**
Patient Health Questionnaire two/nine-question tools (PHQ-2/PHQ-9)	Depression screening	If PHQ-2 positive ($\geq$3), then follow up
General Anxiety Disorder, two/seven -question tool (GAD-2/GAD-7))	Anxiety screening	If GAD-2 positive (>3), then follow up
Beck Depression/Anxiety Inventory (BDI-II/BAI)	Depression/ Anxiety screening	
Somatic Symptom Scale (SSS-8)	Somatic symptom burden from stress and anxiety	Based on PHQ-15
Depression and Anxiety Assessment Test (DAAT)	Depression and anxiety	Nedley Health, $$ for online assessment; also helps determine causes in individual patients, e.g. addiction, nutritional, social, etc.

Table 11-5. DSM-V Criteria for Depression, Anxiety, and PTSD

Condition	Major Criteria	Minor Criteria
Depression	Depressed mood OR anhedonia (loss of interest)	4 of the following: sleep disturbance, psychomotor agitation, fatigue, executive dysfunction, worthlessness or guilt, SI or thoughts of death, part of a bipolar diagnosis
Anxiety	Excessive worry on majority of days for more than 6 months OR difficult to control worry	3 of the following: sleep disturbance, muscle tension, easily fatigued, restlessness or feeling on edge, muscle tension, irritability, difficulty concentrating or mind going blank
PTSD	Criteria A-C, F-H: Exposure through experiencing or learning of an experience of some trauma or threat. AND Unwanted and persistent memories, flashbacks, reminders, or nightmares. AND Thoughts, feelings, or reminders. AND Developed symptoms from stimulus last more than 1 month and create functional impairment or distress.	Criterion D and E: 2 in each of Group 1 and Group 2 symptoms. Group 1 symptoms: incomplete memory of trauma, overly negative thoughts about oneself or world, exaggerated blame of oneself or others for trauma, negative affect, difficulty experiencing positive affect, decreased interested in doing things, and feeling isolated. Group 2 symptoms: irritability or aggression, risky or destructive behavior, hypervigilance, heightened startle reaction, difficulty concentrating, difficulty sleeping

Table 11-6. Self-Management and Resilience Building Tips

Stress management (11-3)	Integrate interests/hobbies	Meet spiritual needs
Cognitive Behavior Therapy	Keep a gratitude journal	Limit screen time
Time management skills	Community support*	Professional support*

These aren't self-reliance, but still useful for improving mental and emotional health.

Table 11-7. Mindfulness Based Stress Reduction

Origin and goals	Program that was designed by Jon Kabat-Zinn to help someone reduce stress and develop coping strategies for stress
Program Details	9 classes over 8 weeks. Then practice formal mindfulness for 45 min/day, 6 days/week. Then, apply informal mindfulness in day-to-day activities.
If it works	No evidence of harm; no evidence of better than pharmacologic treatment; moderate evidence of improved anxiety, depression, and pain
Impact on neuroplasticity	- Inc activation of L prefrontal cortex (planning, personality, and happiness) - Inc gray matter density in hippocampus/other structures responsible for self-awareness, compassion, and introspection - Reduce gray matter density in **amygdala** - fear/stress
Mindfulness for the clinician	- reduced rumination, improved memory, sustained attention, improved focus, stress reduction, less emotional reactivity, improved cognitive flexibility, higher relationship satisfaction, higher ability to deal w/ conflict - improved mental well-being, including calmness, clarity, and concentration - improved empathy, compassion, counseling skills, quality of life and dec psychological stress -

Table 11-8. Supplements for Mental Health Improvement

Omega-3 fatty acids	5-adenosyl methionine (SAMe)
N-acetyl cysteine (NAC)	Zinc
Folate	Vitamin D
Lavender	Saffron
Saponins	Vitamin B12
Chamomile	Magnesium

Table 11-9. Pharmacologic Stress Management Techniques

SSRI / SNRIs	first line, safe in patients w/ CAD
TCA	in patients who don't tolerate SSRI / SNRIs. In patients w/ CAD is not safe because of potential for QT prolongation and orthostatic hypotension
MAOIs	not first or second line, check compatibility with diet and meds
Referral	MDD, SI, HI, prior suicide attempt, comorbid mood disorder, unclear diagnosis, no improvement w/ treatments you feel comfortable with

Physicians must maintain expert levels of both emotional and cognitive intelligence for patient encounters.

Table 11-10. Optimizing Emotional and Cognitive Intelligence in Clinical Encounters

Why is it important	Positive patient-provider relationship improves emotional well-being for everyone
Maintaining one's emotional well-being	Ensure adequate self-care, adequate self-empathy and self-compassion; avoid burnout, avoid compassion fatigue
Maintaining one's ability to be mindful with patients	Maintain a healthy lifestyle (adequate sleep, proper nutrition, physical activity, healthy recreation, no addictions), don't multi-task, take breaks, downshift if too stressed, prepare for the encounter, establish awareness without identifying (judging), sustain focused attention, be able to understand big picture but also talk details, connect on a human level

CHAPTER 12
POSITIVE PSYCHOLOGY FOR LIFESTYLE MEDICINE

Table 12-1. Definitions

Term	Definition
Achievement	Setting and attainment of goals providing sense of satisfaction and pride
Engagement	Complete absorption in moment, inc through intellect, skill, and emotions
Meaning	Purpose that gives life fulfillment and contentedness
Positive emotions	Emotions that enable/enhance ability to see the good aspects of life
Positive psychology	The study of why certain individuals & groups of any size flourish. It is important to note that it does not minimize misery or the experience of neg emotions but focuses instead on strengths to improve the condition.
Relationships	Positive social connections with other humans, emotionally & physically
Eudaimonia	Concern with purposeful living, with minimal regards to pleasures; a process more than an end state; leads to increased longevity
Hedonia	Concern with pleasurable living and satisfaction of desire; egocentric

The underlying assumption behind this chapter is that people have **personal traits, values, and motives** (some of which are more productive towards LM principles than others) that we as clinicians can identify through awareness and assessment and then **use to provide a more personalized clinical approach** resulting in better health outcomes for the patient while fostering improved emotional well-being.

PERMA: A model used in positive psychology to define its fundamental aspects
- **P**ositive emotions
- **E**ngagement
- **R**elationships
- **M**eaning
- **A**chievement

An example of how to approach a positive psychology question:
QUESTION: Dr. Jaferd has a history of enjoying taking more classes than she needs to in college, engaging with people about their fields of work even if she has no knowledge of them, and making friends with different people that she meets while traveling. She has been feeling down and is wondering if she is depressed. Which of the following activities would you suggest to her that might uplift her:
  a) Volunteer in an animal shelter
  b) Keep a gratitude journal
  c) Engage in deep piety
  d) Write a book

To answer this question, you need to be familiar with the following chart:

Table 12-2. Six Core Virtues and 24 Character Strengths of Positive Psychology

Wisdom and Knowledge	Creativity
	Curiosity
	Open-mindedness
	Love of learning
	Perspective
Courage	Bravery
	Persistence
	Honesty
	Zest
Humanity	Love
	Kindness
	Social Intelligence
Justice	Teamwork
	Fairness
	Leadership
Temperance	Forgiveness
	Modesty
	Prudence
	Self-regulation
Transcendence	Appreciation of beauty and excellence
	Gratitude
	Hope
	Humor
	Religiousness

Ruch, et al. Values in Action Inventory of Strengths (VIA-IS): Adaptation and Validation of the German Version and the Development of a Peer-Rating Form. Journal of Individual Differences. January 2010.

APPROACH TO POSITIVE PSYCHOLOGY EXAMPLE QUESTION:

Step 1: Identify each of her activities as one of the 24 character strengths. Some of them may feel like they fit into multiple areas, choose the best fit.

Taking more classes than she needs to in college may indicate a *love of learning*.

Engaging with people about their fields of work even if she has no knowledge of them demonstrates *curiosity*.

Making friends with different people that she meets while traveling exhibits both *open-mindedness* and *social intelligence*.

Step 2: Determine the predominant core virtue exhibited.

Three of the four character strengths identified fall into the Wisdom and Knowledge core virtue. (See Table 12-2_

Step 3: Determine which answer choice best aligns with one of the character strengths in the matching core virtue.

      a) Volunteer in an animal shelter → Kindness → Humanity
      b) Keep a gratitude journal → Gratitude → Transcendence
      c) Engage in deep piety → Religiousness → Transcendence
      d) Write a book → Creativity → Wisdom and Knowledge

ANSWER:

For this example question, the correct answer choice is **d) *Write a book***.

Table 12-3. How Positive Psychology / Emotional Well-Being Affects Health

a reduction in mortality among elderly people
reduced likelihood of being diagnosed with Alzheimer's
slower rate of cognitive decline
reduced likelihood of having strokes and heart attacks
enhanced likelihood of participating in preventive labs and screening exams
more positive relationships
less inflammatory markers
more adaptivity and recovery from negative stimulation
more insular cortex grey matter volume, leading to higher cortical functioning and more complex processing power

Table 12-4. Lifestyle Modifications That Affect Emotional Well-Being

Nutrition / Diet	Significant associations between food and mood, no causation; in general, more plant-based = better mood; nutritional deficiencies w/ higher rates of mood disorders include folate, vitamin B_{12}, calcium, iron, selenium, zinc, and omega-3 fatty acids
Physical Activity	Exercise helps prevent and treat depression; works synergistically with anti-depressant medications
Sleep	7-9 hours of sleep / better quality of sleep correlated with improved mental health
Stress Reduction	Mindfulness improves stress, which improves coping, in turn improving emotional well-being
Toxic Substances	Substance avoidance leads to greater emotional well-being and less volatility

Connectedness is associated with:
- longevity (among 268 male Harvard students followed over 75 years, social connection was the "single most important predictor of happiness and longevity")
- improved heart rate
- activation of parasympathetic (versus sympathetic) nervous system

Waldinger, R. and Schulz, M. What's Love Got to Do With It? Social Functioning, Perceived Health and Daily Happiness in Married Octogenarians. Psychology and Aging. Vol. 25, No. 2, 422– 431. 2010.

On the other hand, *social media* (potential source for negativity) is associated with:
- increased depression
- poor sleep (nighttime specific use)
- increased anxiety and low self-esteem (particularly when emotionally invested)

Table 12-5. Blue Zones Power 9 Traits

Move Naturally	Wine at 5pm	Right Tribe – close friends
Plant Slant to Diet*	Downshift	Family/Loved Ones First
80% Rule (eat 4/5 of plate)	Purpose	Belong

For longevity, 5 servings of fruits and vegetables is good but more is better. At least half should be vegetables.

CHAPTER 13
KEY STUDIES

These studies have changed over the years, although some have remained constant. Check the updated list from ACLM.

1. Primary care-led weight management for remission of T2DM (DiRECT): an open-label, cluster-randomized trial (Lean et al. 2018 Lancet)

Objectives:
- Investigate whether effective weight management in primary care setting could produce sustained remission of T2DM.

Methods	Intervention/Control	Limitations

Open-label, cluster-randomized trial
 	
49 practice sites
 	
Overweight/obese M/F with diabetes diagnosis within 6y and HbA1c >6
 	
306 individuals recruited
 	
23 intervention/26 control practices
 	
12 months
 	
DiRECT: **Di**abetes, **RE**mission, **C**linical **T**rial
	Intervention:
	  Goal to achieve and maintain 15kg weight loss:
	    Phase 1:
	      - Liquid meal replacement (about <u>800 kcal/day</u>) x3mo
	    Phase 2:
	      - Food reintroduction over 2-8 wks
	      - Monthly visits
	  Antidiabetic and antihypertensive meds held on day 1 and reintroduced as needed in Phase 2
	
	  Physical activity maintained during Phase 1, encouraged to increase during Phase 2 to a sustainable maximum (number of steps)
	
	Control:
	  Best practice care guidelines
		Dropout rate of 25% in intervention group
		
		Incomplete data sets
		
		Some patients considered a success had rescue plans initiated

Results	Take-away

Weight reduction > 15kg
  Rx: 24% (mean weight loss 10kg)
  Co: none (mean weight loss 1kg)
 	
Diabetes remission*
  Rx: 46%
  Co: 4%
 	
Remission only achieved by those who lost weight (higher rates associated with more weight lost; e.g., 86% remission in those who lost >15 kg)
	1. Professionally supported intensive weight program achievable and sustainable
	
	2. Diabetes remission had a dose-dependent relationship with weight lost
	
	3. Nearly 50% diabetes remission
	
	4. Nearly 70% stopped antihypertensives

*Remission defined as HbA1c <6.5% after at least 2 months off antidiabetic meds

2. Intensive Lifestyle Changes for Reversal of Coronary Heart Disease (Ornish et al. 1998 JAMA)

Objectives:
- Feasibility/sustainability of intensive lifestyle changes
- Effects lifestyle changes on risk factors, coronary atherosclerosis, myocardial perfusion, and cardiac events

Methods	Intervention/Control	Limitations
Randomized invitational study; intervention for 1y with added 5y follow-up M/F with angiographically documented coronary atherosclerosis/no MI in past 6 wk Originally 48 patients (1y), reducing to 35 patients (5y)	Intensive lifestyle change (N=20): - Vegetarian diet 10% fat - Moderate aerobic exercise 180 min/wk - Stress management training 1 h/day - Smoking cessation - Group psychosocial support 1 h/wk Control (N=15): Follow PCP advice for healthy lifestyle (results were close to AHA step 2 diet: moderate fat 25% and exercise 3x/wk)	Only 3 females (all in control group) Study powered for 1y, with 13 patients not completing through 5y

Results	Take-away

5y adherence scores were excellent in about 60% of cases
 	
LDL-C:
  Rx: 40% decline (1y) up to 20% (5y) without lipid lowering meds
  Co: 6% decline (1y) up to 20% (5y) with lipid lowering meds in over half
 	
Angina:
  Rx: 91% reduction (1y) and 72% reduction (5y)
  Co: 186% increase (1y) leading to angioplasty for 3 patients, and 36% decline (5y)
 	
Coronary stenosis:
  Rx: Diameter decreased by 1.75% (1y) and 3.1% (5y)
      Relative rates of 4.5% (1y) and 7.9% (5y)
  Co: Diameter increased by 2.3% (1y) and 11.8% (5y)
      Relative rates 5.4% (1y) and 27.7% (5y)
      Secondary analysis of control group:
        - On lipid lowering meds: Increased by 6%
        - No meds: Increased by 19%
 	
Cardiac Events*:
  Rx: 25
  Co: 45 (RR 2.47)
 	
No change in TG, HDL, BP
	1. Primary determinant of change in percent diameter stenosis was adherence to recommend lifestyle changes
	
	2. Reversal of coronary artery stenosis possible (improvement continued for years after acute intervention discontinued)
	
	3. Improvements in LDL-C, angina, acute cardiac events

*Cardiac events-myocardial infarction, coronary angioplasty, coronary artery bypass surgery, cardiac-related hospitalizations, cardiac-related deaths
Note: Rx = Treatment group   Co = Controls

3. Comparison of Atkins, Ornish, Weight Watchers, and Zone Diets for Weight Loss and Heart Disease Risk Reduction (Dansinger et al. 2005 JAMA)

Objectives:
- Assess adherence rates for various diets
- Effectiveness for weight loss and cardiac risk factor reduction

Methods	Intervention/Control	Limitations

Randomized controlled trial, single center
 	
Overweight/obese M/F with at least 1 cardiac RF:
  SBP >145 mm Hg
  DBP >90 mm Hg
  Fasting glucose >110 mg/dL
  Total cholesterol >200 mg/dL
  LDL >130 mg/dL
  HDL <40 mg/dL
  TG >150 mg/dL
  On meds for HT, dyslipidemia, or DM
 	
160 patients assigned to 4 groups; 2 mo maximum effort, followed by patient choice of adherence level; 1y follow-up
	Group diet classes 1hr (4x/2mo)
	
	All encouraged to take MVI, 60 min exercise/wk, avoid commercial support services
	
	Atkins goal: <20g carb/day with gradual increase to 50g/day
	
	Zone goal: 40% carb, 30% fat, 30% protein
	
	Weight Watchers goal: 24-32 points daily (about 1200-1600 calories)
	
	Ornish goal: Low fat (10%) vegetarian diet
	
	Outcomes assessed at baseline, 2 mo, 6 mo, 12 mo
		High attrition rate (42% by 12 mo), worse for Atkins/Ornish
		
		Self-reported dietary intake/adherence
		
		Does not evaluate long-term safety risks
		
		Fiber intake low in all (over-reported adherence to Ornish?)
		
		(Not designed to determine best diet)

Results	Take-away

Poor adherence
  - Only 25% a clinically meaningful adherence level
 	
Weight loss:
  - In all groups: 25% sustained a 5% weight loss, 10% sustained a 10% weight loss
  - Association between adherence and weight loss
  - Weight loss associated with decreased HDL, CRP, and insulin
 	
Risk Factors:
  LDL reduced (except Atkins)
  HDL increased (except Ornish)
  LDL/HDL ratio decreased in all by about 10%
  CRP reduced (except Zone)
  Fasting insulin reduced (except Atkins)
 	
No changes in TG, blood pressure, or fasting glucose at 1y.
Caloric intake was not significantly different between diets.
Change in prescription medication was not significantly different between diets (exclusion of patients who initiated cholesterol meds did not change statistical significance of LDL/HDL changes)
	1. Adherence level (rather than diet type) was key determinant of clinical benefits
	
	2. Poor sustainability and adherence levels in all groups resulted in modest weight loss and reduction of cardiac risk factors

4. Effect of Low-Fat versus Low-Carbohydrate Diet on 12-month Weight Loss in Overweight Adults and the Association with Genotype Pattern or Insulin Secretion (Gardner et al. 2018 JAMA)

Objectives:
- Effectiveness of healthy low-fat vs. low-carbohydrate diet on weight loss
- Investigate if genotype pattern or insulin secretion are related to dietary effects on weight loss

Methods	Intervention/Control	Limitations
Randomized controlled trial, parallel group design	Small group sessions average 2x/mo (more frequent in first few months)	20% dropout rate
Overweight/obese M/F	Healthy low-fat goal (50% carb, 30% fat, 20% protein)	Not randomized according to genotype or insulin secretion
Excluded diabetes, HTN, CVD, renal or liver disease, or on meds for those disorders	Healthy low-carb goal (30% carb, 45% fat, 25% protein)	Missing data on initial enrollees
609 adults randomized to low-fat or low-carb diet	Reduced fat or carb to 20g/d for first 8 wks, then slowly added back weekly until lowest sustainable level reached	Limited accuracy of self-reported diet assessments and physical activity tools
12 months	Both groups: No caloric restriction	Rapidly advancing techniques for evaluation of genetic/metabolic phenotypes
DIETFITS: Diet Intervention Examining The Factors Interacting with Treatment Success	Maximize vegetables; minimize sugars, refined flours and trans fats; focus on whole foods Physical activity guidelines 150 min/wk Emotional awareness emphasized	

Results	Take-away
Adherence was good; met macro goals for each group Weight loss: - No difference between diet groups (avg 5-6kg lost), genotype matched or insulin levels Genotype: - Low carb group-32% had low carb responsive SNP, 38% low fat - Low fat group-43% had low fat responsive SNP, 27% low carb No difference in energy/caloric intake, although both had reduction of 500-600 kcal/d Secondary outcomes: - Improvement in both groups (no between group difference) for - BMI, body fat percentage, waist circumference, lipid profiles, blood pressure, insulin, and glucose levels - Low fat favored lower LDL; low carb favored higher HDL and lower TG	1. No significant difference in weight change between healthy low-fat or healthy low-carbohydrate diet 2. Neither genotype nor baseline insulin secretion was associated with dietary effects on weight loss

5. Fasting-Mimicking Diet Promotes Ngn3-Driven Beta-cell Regeneration to Reverse Diabetes (Cheng, Longo et al. 2017 Cell)

Objectives:
- Determine if cycles of FMD can promote the generation of insulin producing beta cells
- Investigate mechanisms responsible for these effects

Methods	Intervention/Control	Limitations
Mice group (T1DM and T2DM) Human pancreatic islet cells (ex vivo) Healthy human adults (serum collection only)	Mouse: Fasting mimicking diet (FMD): low calorie, low carb, low protein, high fat Phase 1: - 50% of standard daily intake on day - 10% on days 2-4 Phase 2: - Ad lib chow for 10 days until next FMD cycle Human (5 days): Plant based (45% carb, 45% fat, 10% protein) meals and snacks provided - Day 1: 1100 kcal - Day 2-5: 720 kcal	Non-human study

Results	Take-away
Mice: FMD cycles rescued mice from late-stage T2DM by restoring insulin secretions and reducing insulin resistance (plasma blood glucose levels normalized) FMD cycles induced beta cell regeneration to reverse beta cell loss (T2DM) FMD T1DM alleviated hyperglycemia and insulin deficiency, reversed (induced) beta cell loss FMD reduced cytokines associated with beta cell damage and increased cytokines associated with beta cell regeneration FMD in non-DM mice promotes a decrease in number of differentiated cells, followed by induction of transitional cells and major increases in the proliferation and number of insulin-generating beta cells FMD promoted a gene expression profile like that observed during embryonic development FMD induced beta cell regeneration is Ngn3 dependent Ex vivo human islet cells: In healthy and T1DM islet cells exposed to serum of FMD treated subjects, there was a trend for induction of expression of Sox2, Ngn3, and insulin (IGF-1 reversed the Sox2 and insulin expression)	1. FMD reverses IDDM and NIDDM phenotypes in mouse models (restores insulin secretion and glucose homeostasis) 2. FMD promotes reprogramming of pancreatic cells to restore insulin generation in islets from IDDM humans

6. Reversal of T2DM: normalization of beta cell function in association with decreased pancreas and liver triacylglycerol (Lim et al. 2011 Diabetologia)

Objectives:
- Investigate if acute negative energy balance alone can reverse beta cell failure and insulin resistance
- Quantify the change in fat content of pancreas and liver

Methods	Intervention/Control	Limitations
Cohort (prospective observational) Adult overweight/obese patients with diabetes diagnosis for <4y 11 patients (9 M, 2 F) Control group (weight matched w/o diabetes) for comparison	Intervention: - Liquid meal replacement (<u>600 kcal/d</u>) - 3 daily servings of non-starchy vegetables - Encouraged water - Maintain baseline physical activity Assessments at 1, 4, 8 wks Follow-up (off diet) at 12 wks Control: - No change	Small size Short term outcomes Difficulty in measuring islet intracellular fatty acid content Some controls had elevated liver fat despite no metabolic abnormality

Results	Take-away
Plasma glucose decreased and was not significantly different than control group after 1 week and was maintained through week 8 HbA1c decreased and was not significantly different from control group at week eight Basal hepatic glucose production decreased to normal levels by wk one and was not significantly different than control at week eight Hepatic triacylglycerol content decreased to control levels by week 1 and was declined to normal/non-obese range by week 8 (average 70% reduction of fat) Pancreatic triacylglycerol content decreased significantly in diabetic group by eight wks Beta cell sensitivity to glucose: - First phase insulin response increased and by eight wks was not significantly different than control - Maximal insulin response surpassed controls by eight wks Total cholesterol and TGL decreased over eight wks Average weight lost was 15kg At 12 wk followup: - three patients had recurrence of diabetes - Mean weight gain: 3kg - Most parameters were unchanged except modest increase in fasting plasma glucose	1. Dietary energy restriction alone led to normalization of beta cell function and hepatic insulin sensitivity in early stage NIDDM 2. Liver and pancreatic fat decreased 3. There was a succession from early change in hepatic insulin sensitivity to a slower change in beta cell function

7. Cardiovascular Effects of Intensive Intervention in T2DM (The Look AHEAD Research Group 2013 NEJM)

Objectives:
- Investigate whether intensive lifestyle intervention for weight loss would decrease cardiovascular morbidity and mortality in overweight or obese patients with diabetes

Methods	Intervention/Control	Limitations
Randomized clinical trial, 16 centers Overweight/obese patients with T2DM (N=5145) 13y follow-up (stopped early at 9y due to futility) AHEAD: **A**ction for **HEA**lth in **D**iabetes Secondary outcome: - Rate of DM remission	Intervention: - Moderate exercise (175 min/week) - Liquid meal replacement and caloric restriction (1200-1800 kcal/day and decreased fat intake) with goal of >7% weight loss - Group/individual counseling x1y, then phone contact 2x/mo Control: - 3 group sessions/y on nutrition/physical activity - Social support in years 1-4, then once a year	Focus was caloric restriction, not diet composition Patients enrolled were motivated Patients in intervention group on average did not meet goal weight loss

Results	Take-away
At study end, mean weight loss was 6% in intervention group (did reach 8% at year 1) Most CV risk factors improved, but effect waned with HbA1c and SBP showing most sustained difference No significant difference in cardiovascular event occurrences (individually or composite) between groups	1. Intensive lifestyle intervention focused on weight loss did not reduce the rate of cardiovascular events in overweight/obese adults with T2DM 2. However, intervention group had meaningful reductions in weight, HbA1c and higher rates of partial remission in first four years

8. Reduction in the Incidence of T2DM with Lifestyle Intervention or Metformin (Diabetes Prevention Program Research Group 2002 NEJM)

Objectives:
- Does a lifestyle intervention or treatment with metformin prevent or delay the onset for diabetes?
- Do these two interventions differ in effectiveness?
- Do their effects differ according to age, sex, race, or ethnicity?

Methods	Intervention/Control	Limitations
Randomized clinical trial, 27 centers >25yo, M/F, overweight or obese, fasting glucose between 95-125 mg/dL, OGTT 140-199 mg/dL (N=3234) Follow-up avg 2.8y (range 1.8-4.6y)	Standard lifestyle + metformin (850mg BID) (standard recommendations were given in written form and an annual 30 min individual session) Standard lifestyle + placebo BID Intensive lifestyle: - Goal of >7% weight loss through low-calorie, low-fat diet - Moderate physical activity (150 min/wk) - A 16-lesson curriculum on lifestyle over first 6 months, then monthly meetings with case manager A fourth group (on troglitazone) was discontinued early due to concern for liver toxicity	Self-reported physical activity and nutrition questionnaires yearly Caloric intake not held constant (intensive lifestyle group had about double calorie reduction) Placebo group more adherent than metformin group Not meant to evaluate relative contributions of diet, physical activity, or weight loss

Results	Take-away
Incidence of diabetes/100 person-yrs: - Placebo: 11 - Metformin: 7.8 - Intensive lifestyle: 4.8 Compared to placebo: - Metformin reduced incidence by 31% (NNT 14) - Intensive lifestyle reduced incidence by 58% (NNT 7) Compared to metformin: - Intensive lifestyle reduced incidence by 39% Intensive lifestyle group adherence: - 50% met weight loss goal by 24wks, down to 38% at last follow-up - Physical activity goal met by 74% at 24 wks, down to 58% at last follow-up Results similar across sex, race, ethnicity; at least as effective in older patients as in younger patients	1. Intensive lifestyle changes and metformin are both highly effective at delaying or preventing T2DM, lifestyle particularly so

9. Effects of Dietary Portfolio of Cholesterol-Lowering Foods vs. Lovastatin on Serum Lipids and C-Reactive Protein (Jenkins et al. 2003 JAMA)

Objectives:
   - Determine effectiveness of a diet rich in cholesterol lowering foods compared to statins

Methods	Intervention/Control	Limitations
Randomized clinical trial 46 adults (25 M and 21 postmenopausal F) with hyperlipidemia 1 month	Group 1: Vegetarian diet very low in saturated fat Group 2: Same diet as Group 1, plus 20mg daily lovastatin Group 3 (Portfolio foods): Vegetarian diet high in plant sterols (margarine), soy protein, viscous fibers (oats, barley, psyllium), almonds; eggs and butter to balance saturated fat in Groups 1 and 2	Food was provided; only 40% found portfolio diet acceptable (some question as to ease of adherence when independent) Small group size

Results	Take-away
LDL reduced by similar amounts in statin (31%) and portfolio groups (28%); greater than control group, but not different from each other CRP reduced by similar amounts in statin (33%) and portfolio groups (28%); greater than control group, but not significantly different from each other Framingham CHD risk score reduced by similar amounts in statin and portfolio groups (mostly due to effect on lipids) Blood pressure and weight loss not significantly different	1. Low saturated fat diet with added portfolio foods reduces LDL-C and CRP comparably to statin

10. Changes in prostate gene expression in men undergoing an intensive nutrition and lifestyle intervention (Ornish et al. 2008 PNAS)

Objectives:
- Examine relationship between comprehensive diet and lifestyle changes and gene expression in the prostate

Methods	Intervention/Control	Limitations
Prospective pilot clinical intervention study 30 M with indolent low risk prostate cancer (no surgery or radiation) GEMINaL Gene Expression Modulation by Intervention with Nutrition and Lifestyle	Intervention: 1. Vegetarian whole food diet 10% fat with supplements (soy, fish oil, vit E, selenium, vit C) 2. Moderate aerobic exercise 180min/wk 3. Stress management training 1h/day 4. Group psychosocial support 1h/wk Prostate needle biopsy at baseline and 3 mo (paired mRNA samples with real time PCR)	Small group/short term No control (baseline biopsy acted as comparison) Variability of biopsy sample Only 30% of biopsies contained tumor cells Food provided (real world adherence?)

Results	Take-away
Response evaluated in normal tissues given that <30% biopsies contained tumor Gene expression: 48 genes up regulated 453 genes down regulated (RAS oncogenes-tumorigenesis and protein metabolism) Weight, abdominal obesity, blood pressure and lipid profile improved in all	Prostate gene expression in normal prostate tissue may be modulated by intensive diet and lifestyle changes

11. Effect of Comprehensive Lifestyle Changes on Telomerase Activity and Telomere Length in Men with Biopsy-Proven Low-Risk Prostate Cancer: 5-Year Follow-up of a Descriptive Pilot Study (Ornish et al. 2013 Lancet Oncol)

Objectives:
- Investigate effect of intensive lifestyle changes on telomere length

Methods	Intervention/Control	Limitations
Prospective clinical intervention study 25 M with indolent low-risk prostate cancer (no surgery or radiation) - 10 controls 5y follow-up on a 3mo pilot study that showed increase in telomerase activity (chromosome elongation)	Intervention: - Vegetarian whole food diet: 10% fat with supplements (soy, fish oil, vitamin E, selenium, vitamin C) - Moderate aerobic exercise (180min/wk) - Stress management training (1h/day) - Group psychosocial support (1h/wk) - Weekly 4hr meetings 3x/mo, then optional 2x/mo Control: - Surveillance only	Small group Short term Nonrandomized Telomere length and telomerase activity measured in peripheral blood samples, not prostate tissue

Results	Take-away
Relative telomere length increased 0.06T/S units in lifestyle group, compared to a decrease in control group by 0.03T/S units - When patients who had treatment for cancer were excluded, the effect was slightly lower Favorable lifestyle adherence dose response Age independently predictive of telomere shortening Telomerase activity decreased in both groups (no difference between groups) PSA concentration increased in both groups (no difference between groups)	1. Lifestyle intervention was associated with significant increases in relative telomere length in men with early-stage prostate cancer, compared to surveillance alone

12. Percutaneous coronary angioplasty compared with exercise training in patients with stable coronary artery disease: A randomized trial (Hambrecht et al. 2004 Circulation)

Objectives:
- Compare exercise training with percutaneous coronary intervention as first line strategy for stable coronary artery disease

Methods	Intervention/Control	Limitations

Randomized controlled trial
 	
Adult M <70yo with stable CAD and 1 coronary artery stenosis >75% (N=101)
 	
Eligible patients had angina (class I-III) and documented myocardial ischemia
 	
12 months
	Angioplasty group (50):
	- PCI performed on average 14 days after randomization
	- ASA throughout study, clopidogrel x4wks after PCI
	
	Exercise group (51):
	- Bicycle ergometer:
	  o First 2 wks in hospital, 6x/day for 10 min each at 70% max HR (symptom free).
	  o Then at home 20 min/day at 70% max HR
	- Weekly 60 min group aerobics class
	
	In both, coronary angiography was performed at baseline and 12 months
		Did not use drug-eluting stents, which could have changed outcome
		
		Small group

Results	Take-away

47 in each group completed baseline and follow-up angiography
  o Compliance high (70%) in exercise group
 	
Composite acute ischemic event*-free survival 88% in exercise group, vs. 70% in PCI group (*relative rate 26%*)
  o NNT=5
 	
Angina decreased significantly in both groups
- Cost to improve angina 1 unit (in CCS classification), including cost of rehospitalization or reintervention
  o ~ $7,000 for PCI
  o ~ $3,400 for exercise
 	
Ischemic threshold improved in both groups, but maximal exercise tolerance improved only in exercise group
 	
Hospitalization and revascularization lower in exercise group
 	
VO_2 max (oxygen uptake at peak exercise/ischemic threshold) increased by 16% in exercise group (no significant change in PCI group)
	1. In patients with stable CAD and a coronary stenosis amenable to PCI, a 12-month exercise program resulted in a higher event-free survival rate
	
	2. PCI and exercise were equally effective at relieving angina, but only the exercise group had higher exercise capacity and maximal oxygen uptake
	
	3. Exercise intervention was more cost-effective (half the cost of PCI)

*Events included death from cardiac cause, resuscitation after cardiac arrest, nonfatal MI, cerebrovascular accident, CABG, PTCA of target lesion or other lesions, hospitalization due to worsening angina
Note: NNT = Number Needed to Treat

Made in the USA
Las Vegas, NV
17 December 2024

14531063R00070